New Directions in Rational Emotive Behaviour Therapy

New Directions in Rational Emotive Behaviour Therapy brings together leading figures from the world of Rational Emotive Behaviour Therapy (REBT), both as a testament to the work of Albert Ellis and as a reminder of the vibrancy and vigour of the approach.

The chapters in this book, taken together, show that REB therapists are open to broader developments in the fields of counselling and psychotherapy in general and can also contribute to these developments. The book introduces REBT to readers who are more familiar with CBT and locates REBT within the broader fields of CBT and modern psychotherapy.

The book will interest REBT and CBT therapists and more broadly it will interest those in the helping professions wishing to explore what REBT can currently offer them and how this approach can be practiced.

Windy Dryden, Ph.D., is Emeritus Professor of Psychotherapeutic Studies at Goldsmiths University of London and is an international authority on Rational Emotive Behaviour Therapy (REBT). He has worked in psychotherapy for over 45 years and is the author and editor of over 250 books.

New Directions in Rational Emotive Behaviour Therapy

Edited by Windy Dryden

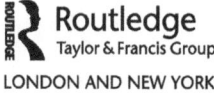
Routledge
Taylor & Francis Group

LONDON AND NEW YORK

First published 2022
by Routledge
2 Park Square, Milton Park, Abingdon, Oxon OX14 4RN

and by Routledge
605 Third Avenue, New York, NY 10158

Routledge is an imprint of the Taylor & Francis Group, an informa business

British Library Cataloguing-in-Publication Data
A catalogue record for this book is available from the British Library

Library of Congress Cataloging-in-Publication Data
Names: Dryden, Windy, editor.
Title: New directions in rational emotive behaviour therapy / edited by Windy Dryden.
Description: Milton Park, Abingdon, Oxon ; New York, NY: Routledge, 2022. |
Includes bibliographical references and index. |
Identifiers: LCCN 2021015439 (print) | LCCN 2021015440 (ebook) |
ISBN 9780367533632 (hardback) | ISBN 9780367533601 (paperback) |
ISBN 9781003081593 (ebook)
Subjects: LCSH: Rational emotive behavior therapy. | Psychotherapy.
Classification: LCC RC489.R3 N49 2022 (print) |
LCC RC489.R3 (ebook) | DDC 616.89/14–dc23
LC record available at https://lccn.loc.gov/2021015439
LC ebook record available at https://lccn.loc.gov/2021015440

ISBN: 978-0-367-53363-2 (hbk)
ISBN: 978-0-367-53360-1 (pbk)
ISBN: 978-1-003-08159-3 (ebk)

DOI: 10.4324/9781003081593

Typeset in Sabon
by Newgen Publishing UK

This book is dedicated to the memory of Arthur Freeman (1942–2020).

Contents

Notes on the editor

Windy Dryden, Ph.D., is Emeritus Professor of Psychotherapeutic Studies at Goldsmiths University of London, and is a Fellow of the British Psychological Society. He has authored or edited more than 250 books, including the second edition of *Reason to Change: A Rational Emotive Behaviour Therapy (REBT) Workbook* (Routledge, 2022) and the third edition of *Rational Emotive Behaviour Therapy: Distinctive Features* (Routledge, 2021). In addition, he edits 21 book series in the area of counselling, psychotherapy and coaching, including the *CBT Distinctive Features* series (Routledge). His major interests are in rational emotive behavior therapy and CBT; single session interventions; the interface between counselling and coaching; pluralism in counselling and psychotherapy; writing short, accessible self-help books for the general public and demonstrating therapy live in front of an audience.

Major affiliation: Goldsmiths University of London

ORCiD identifier: https://orcid.org/0000-0001-5819-749X

Notes on contributors

Damla E. Aksen is a clinical psychology doctoral student at SUNY Binghamton. She has worked in interdisciplinary psychology labs that focused on perception, development, and evolutionary perspectives. As a doctoral student, she has been studying impulsivity, dissociation, mindfulness, emotion dysregulation, and their interrelations. Her current research focuses on clarifying the relations among working memory, emotion dysregulation, dissociation, and impulsivity, and on investigating the effect of each variable on state impulsivity.

Major affiliation: Binghamton University

ORCiD identifier: https://orcid.org/0000-0001-9727-1816

Michal Clayton, B.A., is a doctoral student in clinical psychology at Teachers College, Columbia University, where she works with Dr. Douglas Mennin to investigate the pathophysiology and treatment of distress disorders through the lens of emotion regulation. Her primary research interests involve mechanisms of change in cognitive behavioral treatments for comorbid mood and anxiety disorders. As a doctoral trainee, Ms. Clayton is developing a research program to investigate emotion regulatory strategies at different levels of cognitive elaboration, both as mediators of efficacy in emotion regulation therapy (ERT) and in relation to other psychological variables, such as emotional intensity. She also regularly treats worried and ruminative clients using the ERT framework as part of her clinical training.

Major affiliation: Department of Counseling and Clinical Psychology Teachers College, Columbia University, New York

ORCiD identifier: https://orcid.org/0000-0002-1037-4001

Daniel David, Ph.D., Professor of Clinical Cognitive (Neuro)sciences, is Director of Research and Diplomate/Supervisor at the Albert Ellis Institute (AEI), New York, USA, and president/director of the International Institute for the Advanced Studies of Psychotherapy and Applied Mental Health. He is also a supervisor in the Academy of Cognitive and Behavioral Therapies. After his graduate (Babeş-Bolyai University) and postgraduate (Icahn School of Medicine at Mount Sinai) studies, he got a professorship position at the Babeş-Bolyai University, Cluj-Napoca, Romania, and an adjunct professorship position at the Icahn School of Medicine at Mount Sinai, New York, USA. He is one of the world leaders in promoting the evidence-based approach in clinical psychology/psychotherapy and technology-based clinical psychology/psychotherapy.

Major affiliation: Babeş-Bolyai University/Icahn School of Medicine at Mount Sinai

ORCiD identifier: https://orcid.org/0000-0002-0088-5641

Oana Alexandra David, Ph.D., is Associate Professor in the Department of Clinical Psychology and Psychotherapy at Babeş-Bolyai University and director of the following university based services units: Babeş-Bolyai-PsyTech Psychology Clinic and International Coaching Institute. She is also chief editor of the journal *Evidence-Based Psychotherapies* and member of the editorial board of the *Journal of Rational Emotive and Cognitive Behavioral Therapies*. She is founding president of the International Association of Cognitive Behavioral Coaching and international board member of the International Centre for Coaching Psychology Research, UK. Her research is focused on the efficacy of technology based tools for the prevention of emotional disorders in youth and adults. Based on the research projects she has directed, she developed the following therapeutic technology based tools: the PsyPills app for stress management, the REThink therapeutic game, the online Rational and Positive Parenting Program and the roboRETMAN therapeutic mechatronic device for children.

Major affiliation: Department of Clinical Psychology and Psychotherapy, The International Institute for the Advanced Studies of Psychotherapy and Applied Mental Health, Babeş-Bolyai University, Cluj-Napoca, Romania

ORCiD identifier: https://orcid.org/0000-0001-8706-1778

Raymond DiGiuseppe, Ph.D., received his Bachelor's degree from Villanova in 1971 and his Ph.D. from Hofstra University in 1975, followed by a two-year fellowship with Albert Ellis. Ray was elected a fellow of APA divisions Clinical, School, Psychotherapy, and Family Psychology. He has published extensively on REBT and CBT and on anger as a clinical problem. His works include *Understanding Anger Disorders* and the *Anger Disorders Scale* and the *Anger Regulation and Expression Scale*. He is Professor of Psychology at St. John's University and Director of Education at the Albert Ellis Institute. He has served as president of the Association of Behavioral and Cognitive Therapies and the Society for the Advancement of Psychotherapy (Division 29 of the American Psychological Association). He has worked at the Albert Ellis Institute advancing and promoting REBT for 45 years and has trained psychotherapists in REBT from all over the world.

Major affiliation: St. John's University, New York City, and the Albert Ellis Institute

ORCiD identifier: https://orcid.org/0000-0003-2206-6361

David M. Fresco, Ph.D., is Professor of Psychiatry and Research Professor at the Institute for Social Research (ISR). His program of research adopts an affective neuroscience perspective to conduct basic, translational, and treatment studies of anxiety and mood disorders, particularly distress disorders, incorporating methodologies including functional neuroimaging (fMRI and EEG), peripheral psychophysiology, and serum markers (e.g., inflammation, neurodegeneration). Another facet of Dr. Fresco's research has focused on the development of treatments informed by affective and contemplative neuroscience findings that incorporate mindfulness meditation and other practices derived from Buddhist mental training exercises. Much of his current and recent NIH-funded research has focused on examining neurobehavioral mechanisms and efficacy of mindfulness-enriched treatments for chronic illnesses, and the role of emotion regulation strategies in everyday life to reduce distress.

Major affiliation: University of Michigan, Ann Arbor, MI, USA

ORCiD identifier: https://orcid.org/0000-0001-6736-3912

Irving Kirsch, Ph.D., is Associate Director of the Program in Placebo Studies at the Harvard Medical School and Emeritus Professor of Psychology at the University of Hull (UK) and the University of Connecticut (USA).

He has published 10 books, more than 275 articles, and 40 book chapters on placebo effects, antidepressant medication, hypnosis, and suggestion. He originated the concept of response expectancy. His book *The Emperor's New Drugs: Exploding the Antidepressant Myth* has been published in English, French, Italian, Japanese, Turkish, and Polish, and was shortlisted for the prestigious Mind Book of the Year award. It was the topic of a *60 Minutes* segment on CBS and a five-page cover story in *Newsweek*. In 2015, the University of Basel (Switzerland) awarded Irving Kirsch an Honorary Doctorate in Psychology. In 2019, the Society for Clinical and Experimental Hypnosis honored him with their "Living Human Treasure Award."

Major affiliation: Harvard Medical School

ORCiD identifier: https://orcid.org/0000-0002-1215-4061

Steven Jay Lynn, Ph.D., is Distinguished Professor of Psychology at the State University of New York at Binghamton, the Director of the Clinical Psychology Program, and the former Director of the Psychological Clinic at Binghamton University. He is the author or editor of more than 400 publications on psychotherapy, psychopathology, consciousness, memory, trauma, and hypnosis. Professor Lynn is the inaugural editor of *Psychology of Consciousness: Theory, Research, and Practice (APA)* and recipient of the Indiana University Department of Psychological and Brain Sciences Lifetime Achievement Alumni Award, the Chancellor's Award of the State University of New York for Scholarship and Creative Activities, and awards from the American Psychological Association. His research has been funded by the National Institute of Mental Health and the Ohio Department of Mental Health. He has consulted as an expert witness on hypnosis and memory on a national and international basis, and his work is frequently featured in media venues.

Major affiliation: Binghamton University (SUNY)

ORCiD identifier: https://orcid.org/0000-0002-4493-7810

Walter J. Matweychuk, Ph.D., is a practicing psychologist at the Perelman School of Medicine at the University of Pennsylvania. He also trains doctoral students in Rational Emotive Behavior Therapy. He is an adjunct professor at New York University's Steinhardt School, where he teaches CBT to graduate students of applied psychology. He maintains a private practice in Philadelphia. He is co-author, with Windy Dryden, of

Overcoming Your Addictions and *Rational Emotive Behavior Therapy: A Newcomer's Guide.* He has served as a subject matter expert on a CBT skills classroom project developed for the United States Navy. Visit his website at REBTDoctor.com to join his Intermittent Reinforcement email list and obtain an invitation to attend his weekly REBT Zoom Conversation hour. He can be contacted on rebtdoctor@gmail.com.

Major affiliation: University of Pennsylvania, Perelman School of Medicine

ORCiD identifier: https://orcid.org/0000-0003-4918-4253

Douglas S. Mennin, Ph.D., is a Professor of Clinical Psychology at Teachers College, Columbia University. His work is focused on elucidating the chronically busy mind. He has been most interested in examining how people fail to effectively manage their emotions, particularly when people conceptualize the future and past, and has conducted numerous studies of the basic psychological and physiological mechanisms of chronic anxiety and depression, most recently examining how brief, cost effective, interventions can demonstrate brain and body change and how this change accounts for how people get better. In collaboration with David Fresco, he has developed emotion regulation therapy (ERT), which is an integrative mind–body psychotherapy that draws from contemporary approaches as well as affect science and neuroscience. Outcome findings have been promising, as have the preliminary identification of a number of cognitive, physiological, and neural mechanisms that may help explain how the therapy is effective.

Major affiliation: Teachers College, Columbia University

ORCiD identifier: https://orcid.org/0000-0003-3654-8070

Andrei C. Miu, Ph.D., is Professor of Cognitive Neuroscience and Behavioral Genetics at the Department of Psychology, Babeş-Bolyai University, and the Founding Director of the Cognitive Neuroscience Laboratory, one of the leading research groups in the field of cognitive and affective science in Romania. His research has focused on emotion and emotion regulation, including emotion-linked cognitive biases in decision making, attention and memory; autonomic and neuroendocrine processes in emotion and emotion regulation; gene-environment interactions in emotion; emotion regulation and risk of anxiety and depression.

Major affiliation: Cognitive Neuroscience Laboratory, Department of Psychology, Babeș-Bolyai University, Cluj-Napoca, Romania

ORCiD identifier: https://orcid.org/0000-0002-6459-5010

Diana-Mirela Nechita, Ph.D., is currently Senior Assistant Professor within the Department of Clinical Psychology and Psychotherapy, Faculty of Psychology and Sciences of Education, Babeș-Bolyai University, Romania, and a fellow of the International Institute for the Advanced Studies of Psychotherapy and Applied Mental Health at Babeș-Bolyai University. She is a clinical psychologist and cognitive-behavioral psychotherapist certified by the Romanian National Board of Psychologists. She is also certified by the Albert Ellis Institute, New York, as an REBT psychotherapist. Her main research interests are in evidence-based psychological interventions, self-conscious emotions, and emotion regulation.

Major affiliation: Babeș-Bolyai University, Department of Clinical Psychology and Psychotherapy

ORCiD identifier: https://orcid.org/0000-0002-0750-8953

Craig P. Polizzi, M.S., is a clinical psychology doctoral student at Binghamton University. He is the graduate research coordinator of the Laboratory of Consciousness, Cognition, and Psychopathology. He has collaborated on randomized controlled trials investigating integrative and complementary interventions for veterans with posttraumatic stress disorder (PTSD). His current research focuses on clarifying the relations among acceptance, mindfulness, emotion regulation, dissociation, and trauma and on elucidating how each functions as a regulatory coping strategy to promote resilience.

Major affiliation: Binghamton University (SUNY)

ORCiD identifier: https://orcid.org/0000-0001-9270-6868

Megan E. Renna, Ph.D., is a Postdoctoral Fellow in the Comprehensive Cancer Center and Institute for Behavioral Medicine Research at the Ohio State University College of Medicine. She received her Ph.D. in clinical psychology from Teachers College, Columbia University, in 2019

under the mentorship of Dr. Doug Mennin and completed her clinical internship at Duke University Medical Center. Her research focuses on identifying emotional, cognitive, behavioural, and biological mechanisms linking psychological distress to poor physical health among healthy adults and cancer survivors. She is also interested in intervention research with a specific emphasis on reducing physical and psychological distress through evidence-based approaches. Dr. Renna currently is funded through a T32 institutional training grant sponsored through the National Cancer Institute.

Major affiliation: The Ohio State University College of Medicine

ORCiD identifier: https://orcid.org/0000-0003-3941-4270

Fiona Sleight, B.A., is a clinical psychology master's student at Binghamton University. She is a researcher in the Laboratory of Consciousness, Cognition, and Psychopathology, and her current research centers around elucidating the concept of ego dissolution and its relation to other constructs, such as dissociation and trauma.

Major affiliation: Binghamton University

ORCiD identifier: https://orcid.org/0000-0002-0470-0173

Phillip E. Spaeth is a third-year doctoral student in the Clinical Psychology program at Teachers College, Columbia University. In 2017, he graduated summa cum laude from the CUNY Baccalaureate for Unique and Interdisciplinary Studies, with a concentration in psychology, philosophy, and Asian wisdom traditions. He has worked with Dr. Douglas Mennin and the research team in the Regulation of Emotion in Anxiety and Depression Lab for the past five years. His research interests are focused on emotion regulation and the dissemination of mechanism-targeted interventions, specifically internet and mobile interventions (IMI). Under the mentorship of Dr. Mennin, Phillip has led a team developing "blended" versions of emotion regulation therapy, which incorporate IMI into treatment with varying levels of therapist support.

Major affiliation: Teachers College, Columbia University

ORCiD identifier: https://orcid.org/0000-0001-5092-0014

Aurora Szentágotai-Tătar, Ph.D., is Professor of Clinical Psychology and Psychotherapy at Babeş-Bolyai University, Cluj-Napoca. She is supervisor of Rational Emotive Behavior Therapy (REBT), certified by the Albert Ellis Institute. She is vice-president of the Romanian Association of Cognitive and Behavioral Psychotherapies, fellow of the Albert Ellis Institute, and of the International Institute for the Advanced Studies of Psychotherapy and Applied Mental Health. Her research interests are related to evidence-based psychological interventions and mechanisms of psychopathology.

Major affiliation: Babeş-Bolyai University, Cluj-Napoca

ORCiD identifier: https://orcid.org/0000-0002-2934-4267

Introduction

Windy Dryden

The chapters in this edited book originated at the Fourth International Congress of Rational Emotive Behavior Therapy, 13–15 September 2019, in Cluj-Napoca, Transylvania, Romania. This congress, organized by Dr Daniel David and his fine team at the Department of Psychology at the University of Babeș-Bolyai in Romania, showed the breadth of topics currently under discussion in the CBT community. The chapters in this book demonstrate this breadth and honour the objectives of the Congress. These objectives were to celebrate REBT's 'classical' past, make connections between REBT and the broader world of evidence-based psychotherapy, look at REBT's contribution to various non-clinical fields and reflect on the future of REBT.

The book is divided into three parts. In Part I, *Roots and branches*, I begin in Chapter 1 by introducing REBT to readers who may not be as familiar with it as they are with other CBT approaches. The chapter looks at the roots of REBT, considering the foundations of this stand-alone 'tree'. In Chapter 2, Raymond DiGiuseppe locates REBT within the broader fields of CBT and modern psychotherapy. His chapter considers the connections of the REBT 'tree' with other 'trees' in the 'psychotherapy forest', showing its similarities and differences as the branches of the respective 'trees' reach out towards one another. In Chapter 3, I consider how REBT has 'branched out' to the delivery therapy mode known as single-session therapy and explain why I think that REBT is particularly suited for such brief work.

In Part II, *What REBT practitioners can learn from the wider world of psychotherapy*, noted researchers from areas outside REBT, but who are friendly towards it, show how REBT can be enriched by work done in these areas. Thus, in Chapter 4, research done on emotion regulation is presented and implications for REBT explored. And in Chapters 5 and 6, the lessons that REBT can learn from debates that have long preoccupied the field of psychotherapy research are presented.

In Part III, *The contributions of REBT to coaching, the science of happiness, and as a philosophy of life,* noted scholars in each of the named fields explore what REBT has to offer human endeavour where psychological disturbance is not the primary focus. The results of these explorations are described in Chapters 7–9.

In the closing keynote address at the congress, Arthur Freeman, a well-known cognitive therapist who always maintained contact with his REBT colleagues, gave a paper on REBT's past, present and possible future. It is the only congress address that I have attended where the speaker received a standing ovation. Art was quite ill at the time of the congress and sadly died in August 2020. Oana David and Daniel David prepared the chapter from Art's written notes on his talk and from the recording of the presentation that was made at the time. It appears here as an epilogue in Chapter 10.

Art was held in deep affection by many in the REBT and CBT communities, and I have dedicated this book to his memory. It is fitting that the book should end with a eulogy for Art written by his friend and colleague Mark Gilson.

Part I

Roots and branches

Chapter 1

Rational Emotive Behaviour Therapy

A comprehensive introduction

Windy Dryden

In this chapter, I will begin by considering the evolution of Rational Emotive Behaviour Therapy (REBT) and show how Albert Ellis developed this approach to CBT partly as a result of what he made of his developmental experiences, partly from his interests in philosophy and partly due to his disenchantment with the extant approaches to therapy. I will then outline its distinctive theoretical and practical features. Next, I will briefly consider the research that has been done on the relationship between rigid and extreme attitudes (previously known as irrational beliefs)[1] and psychological disturbance and on the effectiveness of REBT. Finally, I will discuss how REBT has been disseminated to both professionals and the public.

The evolution of REBT

Rational Emotive Behaviour Therapy (REBT) was founded in the mid-1950s by Albert Ellis, with the first publications appearing in 1957 (Ellis, 1957a, 1957b; see also Ellis, 1997). It thus lays claim to be the first formal approach within what is now known as the cognitive-behavioural therapies. In this section, I will consider some of the professional and personal reasons why Ellis developed REBT and some of the influences on his thought. However, first, let me highlight significant name changes to the therapy, which will help the reader understand the historical development of REBT.

From RT to RET to REBT

Originally, in the mid-1950s, Ellis called his approach 'Rational Therapy' (RT) to indicate that it was quite different from the dominant approaches at that time. Thus, he emphasized the cognitive–philosophical aspects of his therapy to indicate its differences from the approaches in the psychoanalytic and humanistic therapy traditions. Because of his keenness to emphasize the role of cognition in people's problems and their remediation, rational

DOI: 10.4324/9781003081593-2

therapy was accused by its critics of neglecting clients' emotions. To make it clear that this was not the case, Ellis (1962) changed the name of his approach to Rational-Emotive Therapy (RET). This name stood until 1993 when, at the prompting of Raymond Corsini, he again changed the name of the approach to Rational Emotive Behaviour Therapy (REBT) in reply to critics who argued that RET neglected clients' behaviours (Ellis, 1993). However, as Ellis (1999) said in a later paper, REBT (and its predecessors) always advocated and incorporated the use of active behavioural methods to encourage clients to practise newly acquired therapeutic insights in their life situation.

As I have said, Ellis originated the first manifestation of REBT, which he called 'Rational Therapy' to emphasize its rational or cognitive features. While working initially as a marriage counsellor (in the early to mid-1940s) and then as a clinical psychologist (in the late 1940s and early 1950s), he became increasingly disenchanted with the traditional humanistic and psychoanalytic therapies of the day, largely because he considered them too passive, ineffective and because they neglected the cognitive modality of human experience. This disenchantment encouraged Ellis to experiment with a variety of other approaches that existed at the time (Ellis, 1955) in a quest to find more effective and efficient therapeutic methods. This search did not bear much fruit.

Philosophical influences

What was more successful was when Ellis went back to his long-standing interest in philosophy and saw the value and relevance of this discipline to the development of effective and efficient therapy that had cognition at its core. In this regard, Ellis was particularly influenced by the writings of Stoic philosophers, such as Epictetus and Marcus Aurelius. The oft-quoted phrase of Epictetus, 'People are disturbed not by things but by their view of things', crystallized Ellis's stance that philosophical factors were more important than psychoanalytic and psychodynamic factors in accounting for psychological disturbance. An up-to-date version of this famous saying, 'People disturb themselves by the rigid and extreme attitudes that they hold towards things', shows the central role given to rigid and extreme attitudes in REBT theory in understanding the roots of psychopathology (Dryden, 2015, 2016).

In addition to the influence of the Stoics, the impact of other philosophers can be discovered in Ellis's writings. Thus, Ellis (1981) was influenced very early on in his career by Kant's writings on both the power and the limitations of cognition and ideation, particularly *The Critique of Pure Reason*. Ellis has argued that REBT is founded upon the logico-empirical methods of science, and in this respect he credited the writings of Popper (1959, 1963) and Reichenbach (1953) as being particularly influential on his efforts to make these philosophical ideas core features of RT, RET and latterly REBT (see below).

REBT is closely identified with the principles of ethical humanism (Russell, 1930, 1965) and also has distinct existential roots. In the latter respect, Ellis (1962) said that he was particularly influenced by the ideas of Paul Tillich (1953). Like other existentialists (e.g., Heidegger, 1949), REBT theorists agree that humans are 'at the centre of their universe (but not of the universe) and have the power of choice (but not of unlimited choice) with regard to their emotional realm' (Dryden & Ellis, 1986: 130). Ellis (1973) wrote on REBT's humanistic foundations and claimed (Ellis, 1984: 23) that it is doubly humanistic in its outlook, in that it: a) helps people maximize their individuality, freedom, self-interest and self-control; and b) helps them live in an involved, committed and selectively loving manner. It thereby strives to facilitate individual and social interest.

The influence of Horney and Adler

Although Ellis claimed that the creation of RT owed more to the work of philosophers than to (pre-1959) psychologists and psychotherapists, he was particularly influenced by the writings of two of the latter. When Ellis originally trained in psychoanalytic methods, he was analysed by a training analyst of the Karen Horney school and the influence of Horney's (1950) ideas on the 'tyranny of the shoulds' influenced Ellis as he developed the central idea in REBT – that rigid attitudes are at the core of psychological disturbance.

Ellis (1973) stated that REBT owes a particular debt to the ideas of Alfred Adler (1927), who held that a person's behaviour springs from their ideas. Adler's concept of the vital role played by feelings of inferiority in psychological disturbance pre-dates Ellis's view that self-esteem problems, based on a global negative evaluation of self, constitute a fundamental human disturbance. REBT also emphasizes the role of social interest in determining psychological health, as did Adler (1964). Other Adlerian influences on REBT are the importance that humans attribute to goals, purposes, values and meanings; the emphasis on active-directive teaching; the employment of a cognitive-persuasive form of therapy; and the teaching method of holding live demonstrations of therapy sessions before an audience.

The influence of general semantics

Ellis's ideas (circa the mid-1970s) were influenced by the work of the general semanticists, who argued that our psychological processes are, to a great extent, determined by our overgeneralizations and by the careless language we employ. Like Korzybski (1933), Ellis held that modification of the errors in our thinking and our language have a marked effect on our emotions and actions. One particular way that Ellis implemented the influence of general semanticists was through the use of e-prime (Bourland, 1965/1966). E-prime is an approach to language that excludes all forms of the verb 'to be' since when this verb is used, we tend to overgeneralize. Thus, if I were to say, 'I am a psychologist,' I tend to identify myself in my mind with this role. However, were I to say, 'I work as a psychologist,' I tend not to make this error. Thus, use of forms of the verb 'to be' oversimplify human beings and are the breeding ground for self-devaluation (e.g. 'I am a failure' rather than 'I failed'). In the mid-1970s, Ellis wrote five books in e-prime, including the bestselling *A New Guide to Rational Living* (Ellis & Harper, 1975), but dropped it soon after because it was too cumbersome. E-prime no longer influences modern REBT

Personal experiences and factors[2]

Having outlined the intellectual roots of Ellis's creation of rational therapy, let me now outline some of the personal influences of its development. It is crucial, in this respect, to realize that the founders of therapy approaches bring themselves as people and their personal experiences to the approaches that they develop. Thus, it is difficult to imagine Albert Ellis developing what is now known as person-centred therapy and difficult to imagine Carl Rogers developing REBT! Ellis dealt with several personal problems and adversities by means of early versions of concepts that appeared later in REBT.

Ellis was the eldest of three children and grew up in a family with a rather self-absorbed mother and absent father. He became self-sufficient quite early on, a characteristic that helped him when he was hospitalized several times between the ages of five and seven. He coped with being in hospital and the paucity of family visits by accepting the reality of the situation and by solving problems in his head.

Ellis was anxious about public speaking and approaching women, but dealt with these issues in ways consistent with later REBT theory and practice. With the former, he resolved to speak in public, but the first time he did so he tripped on the way up to the rostrum to the mirth of his audience. However, he saw that while this was uncomfortable, it was not horrible, and he went on to become one of the best public speakers in the therapy field. He decided to deal with the latter problem by approaching 100 women in the nearby Bronx Botanical Gardens, engaging them in conversation and asking as many as would speak to him on a date. While only one woman agreed to meet him (although she never turned up), Ellis overcame his fear of women because he saw through his repeated practice that nothing awful happened and that he had a number of pleasant conversations. 'Non-awfulizing thinking' and repeated facing up to adversity are two hallmarks of current REBT theory and practice.

RT, as it was known in the early days, met with much disapproval from the field. It would have been easy for Ellis to reconsider his ideas or to keep a low profile, but he did neither, choosing to give as many talks as he could and to distribute his early writings to anyone who was even vaguely interested. Ellis was able to do this, he said, because he did not need approval and because he decided to persist in pursuing what was important to him in the face of adversity.

Throughout his life, Ellis demonstrated high levels of self-discipline in many areas. A good example of this was when he was diagnosed as having Type 1 diabetes at the age of 43. Despite having a very sweet tooth, Ellis immediately followed dietary advice and accepted, without complaining, his daily regime of self-injecting insulin and ongoing monitoring of his blood sugar levels.

These examples show that Ellis adhered in his own life to ideas and practices that were featured in the therapy approach that he developed. He practised what he preached!

Distinctive theoretical features

In this section, I briefly outline the distinctive theoretical features of REBT, while in the following section of the chapter, I will discuss the distinctive practical features of this approach.

Post-modern relativism

REBT theorists espouse post-modern relativism, which is antithetical to rigid and extreme views and holds that, as far as we currently know, there is no absolute way of determining reality. This philosophy stops short of saying that there is no absolute way of determining reality for to do so would violate the central position of post-modernism. Thus, while REBT theorists put forward specific criteria to differentiate rigid and extreme attitudes from flexible and non-extreme attitudes, they hold that these criteria are relative rather than absolute and would be against any such absolute criteria (Dryden, 2015).

REBT's position on human nature

REBT theory has a unique position on human nature. This viewpoint was put forward by Daniel Ziegler (2000), who helped to pioneer a 'nine basic assumptions' approach in personality theory (Hjelle & Ziegler, 1992). Each basic assumption is construed as a seven-point continuum, with two ends and strong (7/1), moderate (6/2) or slight (5/3) leanings towards one end or the other, with a mid-point of 4.

- Freedom (6) – Determinism: REBT holds that people have a moderate amount of freedom to choose the way they respond to external and internal factors.
- Rationality – Irrationality. REBT holds that people occupy the midpoint (4) between these two ends of the continuum. Thus, they are prone to irrationality but capable of rationality.
- Holism (6) – Elementalism. While REBT holds that people can be understood while considering their thinking, behaving and emoting as separate processes, they are better understood when these processes are more accurately considered to be interdependent.
- Constitutionalism (7) – Environmentalism. While most CBT approaches adopt an environmental-focused social learning approach to human disturbance, REBT argues that humans are biologically disposed to disturb themselves about life's adversities; see Ellis (1976) for a full discussion of this point.
- Changeability (6) – Unchangeability. Despite the above, REBT holds that, with committed work, humans are moderately capable of fundamental change over time.
- Subjectivity (7) – Objectivity. REBT has a strong phenomenological emphasis and holds that humans are much more influenced by subjective factors than external, objective factors. Thus, when they do face objective negative events, they more frequently disturb themselves about subjective features of these events more than about the events themselves.
- Proactivity (7) – Reactivity. REBT holds that people are strongly proactive in generating their responses to events. They are not seen as passive responders to external stimuli.
- Homeostasis – Heterostasis. REBT holds that people occupy the midpoint (4) between being motivated to reduce tensions and to maintain inner homeostasis, on the one hand, and being motivated to actualize themselves, on the other hand. Practically, they are helped more effectively with the latter area when they are first helped with the former.
- Knowability – (2) Unknowability. REBT holds that while we can learn much about human affairs, much of human nature is not fully knowable. As Ziegler (2000) noted, this assumption explains why Ellis did not devote much time to formulating an REBT-based personality theory.

REBT's distinctive 'Situational ABC' model

While an *ABC* model for understanding psychological problems can be found in different CBT approaches, REBT uses a distinctive 'Situational *ABC*' model. In this model, the person is deemed to disturb themselves at *C* about an aspect of the 'situation' that they are in (known as the adversity at

A) primarily because they hold a set of rigid and extreme basic attitudes at B (Dryden, 2015). For example:

'Situation'	My boss left a note on my desk asking me to see him as soon as possible.
A (<u>A</u>dversity)	My boss is going to criticize me for something that I have done.
B (Basic <u>Attitude</u>)	(rigid basic attitude) = My boss must not criticize me. (extreme basic attitude) = If my boss criticizes me, that would be terrible.

C (<u>C</u>onsequence)	(emotional) = Anxious
	(behavioural) = Wanting to run away
	        = Takes a sedative before going to see boss
	(cognitive) = My boss will look for ways to fire me.
	      = I will find it hard to get another job because my boss will not give me a good reference.

While the above outlines REBT's 'Situational *ABC*' model of psychological disturbance, the following outlines REBT's model of a psychologically healthy response to the same adversity at *A*. Here, the person is deemed to respond healthily at *C* about the same adversity at *A* largely because they hold a set of flexible and non-extreme basic attitudes at *B* (Dryden, 2015).

'Situation'	My boss left a note on my desk asking me to see him as soon as possible.
A (<u>A</u>dversity)	My boss is going to criticize me for something that I have done.
B (Basic <u>Attitude</u>)	(flexible basic attitude) = I do not want my boss to criticize me, but that does not mean that he must not do so. (non-extreme basic attitude) = If my boss criticizes me, that would be bad, but not terrible.
C (<u>C</u>onsequence)	(emotional) = Concerned (behavioural) = Wanting to face up to what my boss has to say without taking any medication (cognitive) = If my boss is unhappy with something I have done, he will tell me, but he probably will not look for ways to fire me.

This model has several distinctive features:

1. *A* is often inferential in nature. Inferences are deemed to go beyond the data at hand and may be accurate or inaccurate. In the absence of finding

out the 'truth' about what happened, the person may be encouraged to make the 'best bet' given the available data. As will be shown later, in order to identify rigid and extreme attitudes at *B*, practitioners of REBT first encourage their clients to assume temporarily that *A* is true and will work with distorted inferences at *A* after the clients have made progress at changing *Bs* to their flexible and non-extreme alternatives.

2. As shown above, basic attitudes at *B* are the central determining factor of functional and dysfunctional responses at *C* about adversities at *A*.
3. *C* can be emotive, behavioural and cognitive.
4. *ABCs* are best understood within a situational context.

Emphasis on attitudes

Perhaps the central tenet of REBT theory is that rigid attitudes are at the very core of psychological disturbance. Ellis (1994) argued that while what he called irrational beliefs (or what I call 'attitudes') can be rigid or extreme, of the two, it is rigid attitudes that are at the very core of disturbance. Rigid attitudes are often based on preferences but are then transformed into absolutes. Thus, if I hold that it is important to me that you like me, then this is my preference. When I make this preference rigid, I transform it into a demand, thus: 'I want you to like me, and therefore you must do so.' It is important to note that rigid attitudes are often expressed without the preference being made explicit, thus: 'You must like me.'

REBT theorists argue that extreme attitudes are derived from rigid attitudes (Ellis, 1994). Since the theory posits that rigid attitudes are at the very core of disturbance, it follows that other dysfunctional attitudes and distorted cognitions are derived from this rigid core. Extreme attitudinal derivatives are the closest derivatives to this core. REBT theory argues that there are three extreme attitudinal derivatives from rigid attitudes. In the material that follows, I will list and define each extreme attitude and show that it is derived from the person's rigid attitude. These extreme attitudes are known as:

1. *Awfulizing attitudes.* Here the client believes at the time of disturbance that something is so bad that it could not get any worse. For example: 'You must like me, and it would be absolutely awful if you do not.'
2. *Unbearability attitudes.* Here the client holds that they cannot bear the adversity that they are facing or are about to face. For example: 'You must like me, and I could not bear it if you do not.'
3. *Devaluation attitudes.* Here the client gives themself, others or life a global negative evaluation which, at the time, they think defines them, others or life. For example, 'You must like me, and if you do not, I'm not worthy.'

The corollary of the point that rigid attitudes are at the very core of psychological disturbance is that flexible attitudes are at the very core of psychological health. Ellis (1994) argued that while what he called rational attitudes can be flexible or non-extreme, of the two, it is flexible attitudes that are at the very core of psychological health. Flexible attitudes, like rigid attitudes, are often based on preferences, but they are flexible because the person is explicit that they are not rigid. Thus, if I hold that it is important to me that you like me, then this is again my preference. When I keep this preference flexible, I negate the demand, thus: 'I want you to like me, but you do not have to do so.'

REBT theorists also argue that non-extreme attitudes and realistic cognitions are derived from flexible attitudes (Ellis, 1994). Non-extreme attitudinal derivatives are the closest derivatives to this core. REBT theorists argue that there are three non-extreme attitudinal derivatives from flexible attitudes. In the material that follows, I will list and define each non-extreme attitude and show that it is derived from the person's flexible attitude. These non-extreme attitudes are known as:

1. *Non-awfulizing attitudes.* Here the client holds at the time that something is bad, but not the end of the world. For example: 'I want you to like me, but you do not have to do so. It is bad that you do not, but not awful.'
2. *Bearability attitudes.* Here the client holds that it is difficult bearing the adversity that they are facing or are about to face, but that they can bear it and that it is worth it for them to do so. Also, they assert that they are willing to bear the adversity and commit themself to so doing. For example: 'I want you to like me, but you do not have to do so. It would be difficult for me to bear you not liking me, but I can bear it, and it is worth doing so. I am willing to bear you not liking me and will commit myself to do so by facing you.'
3. *Unconditional acceptance attitudes.* Here the client acknowledges that they, others or life are far too complex to merit a global negative evaluation and that such an evaluation does not define them, others or life. For example, 'I want you to like me, but you do not have to do so. I am the same fallible person whether you like me or not.'

REBT's position on negative emotions

REBT theorists distinguish between unhealthy (dysfunctional) negative emotions and healthy (functional) negative emotions. They argue that unhealthy negative emotions and healthy negative emotions are qualitatively different from one another, as unhealthy negative emotions stem from rigid and extreme attitudes toward adversity and healthy negative emotions stem from flexible and non-extreme attitudes about the same adversity (see Dryden, 2015). As such, these distinguishable emotions exist on two separate continua rather than on one single continuum.

For example, anxiety about a threat is underpinned by a rigid and extreme attitude towards the adversity, and its healthy alternative about that same threat is concern, which is underpinned by a flexible and non-extreme attitude. The goal in REBT is not to reduce the intensity of anxiety; rather, it is to help the person to feel concerned rather than anxious about a threat.

How clients create highly distorted inferences: an REBT perspective

When clients discuss their problems with their REB therapists, it sometimes occurs that they report highly distorted inferences. Given the available evidence, it is usually readily apparent to the therapist that such inferences are negatively biased and highly skewed to the negative. However, these inferences seem very real to clients. Examples of such inferences are: 'I am going to have a heart attack', 'Nobody will ever talk to me again' and 'I will always fail and will end up a bag lady'.

REBT theory argues that such inferences are cognitive consequences (at C) of rigid and extreme attitudes (e.g. Dryden, Ferguson & McTeague, 1989). Such inferences are highly distorted because prior related and usually less distorted inferences at A have been processed by the person using their rigid and extreme attitudes at B. However, the client is usually only aware of the highly distorted inference at C as it is very compelling and is usually unaware of both their inference at A and their rigid and/or extreme attitude at B. Here are three examples of this process. Note how the rigid and the extreme processing of A leads to the highly distorted the inference at C. Thus:

A = I am feeling out of control
B = I must gain control immediately
C (cognitive) = If I do not, I will have a heart attack

A = My friends are not talking to me
B = My friends must talk to me, and it is terrible that they are not
C (cognitive) = Nobody will ever talk to me again

A = I may fail a crucial forthcoming exam
B = I must pass this exam, and it will be the end of the world if I do not
C (cognitive) = If I fail, I will always fail and will end up a bag lady

REBT's position on human worth

REBT theory has a unique position on human worth. Actually, it has two positions on this subject, a preferred position and a back-up position. It holds that unchangeable aspects of humans are our:

1. humanness (we are human till we die);
2. complexity (we are too complex to justify a single defining global rating);
3. uniqueness (there will never be another you);
4. fallibility (we have an incurable error-making tendency);
5. changeability (we are constantly in flux).

REBT's preferred position on human worth is that we are neither worth-while nor worthless; rather we just are and we can either choose to accept ourselves as human and as having the above unchangeable aspects or choose not to do so. When we do make this affirmative choice, we can be said to be operationalizing a philosophy of unconditional self-acceptance, which encapsulates REBT's preferred position on human worth.

When clients do not resonate with this position and prefer to regard themselves as having worth, then the best way of doing this without making themselves vulnerable to ego disturbance (see below) is to opt for uncondi-tional self-worth. This back-up position states that I am worthwhile because I am human, complex, unique, fallible and changeable. I could, of course, state that I am worthless because I have these aspects, and this is equally valid for I can neither prove that I am worthwhile nor prove that I am worthless. However, if I want to live healthily and happily, the uncondi-tional self-worth position will facilitate this far more than the unconditional worthlessness position.

According to REBT, the real culprit (apart from unconditional worth-lessness) when it comes to ego disturbance is conditional self-worth. Thus, when a client says, 'I am worthwhile when I am loved, successful, popular and wealthy,' for example, then they disturb themself when they lose any of these factors, and they are vulnerable to disturbance when they have these factors because they can always lose them.

REBT differentiates between ego and discomfort disturbance and health

REBT theorists argue that we have two major domains in which we function as humans: ego and non-ego (here referred to as comfort/discomfort). REBT therefore differentiates between ego disturbance and discomfort disturb-ance, on the one hand, and ego health and discomfort health, on the other.

Ego disturbance in the face of adversity is marked by a rigid attitude and a self-devaluation attitude that is derived from it. For example, a client says,

'I must pass my exam, and I am a failure if I do not.' By contrast, ego health in the face of the same adversity is marked by a flexible attitude and an unconditional self-acceptance attitude that is derived from it. For example, the same client says, 'I would like to pass my exam, but I do not have to do so. If I do not, I am not a failure. I am an unrateable human being who has failed in this respect.'

Discomfort disturbance in the face of adversity is marked by a rigid attitude and an unbearability attitude that is derived from it. For example, a client says, 'I must have the benefits that I will get if I pass my exam, and I could not bear to be deprived of these benefits should I fail.' By contrast, discomfort health in the face of the same adversity is marked by a flexible attitude and a bearability attitude that is derived from it. For example, the same client says, 'I would like to have the benefits that I will get if I pass my exam, but I do not need these benefits. If I fail the exam and am thus deprived of these benefits, then it would be a struggle for me to bear this deprivation. However, I could bear it, it is worth it to me to do so, I am willing to do so, and I commit myself to so doing by...'

There are two other important points worth noting about ego and discomfort disturbance. First, a rigid attitude on its own does not make clear the type of disturbance a person is experiencing. The extreme attitudinal derivative helps to make this clear. Thus, if my rigid attitude is: 'I must retain my autonomy', this attitude, on its own, does not indicate ego or discomfort disturbance. However, if my major extreme attitudinal derivative is: '...and I am a pathetic person if I lose my autonomy', then I am experiencing ego disturbance, whereas if it is: '...and I cannot bear the resultant conditions if I lose my autonomy', then I am experiencing discomfort disturbance.

The second important point is that ego disturbance and discomfort disturbance frequently interact. Thus, I may begin by experiencing ego disturbance and create a disturbed negative emotion such as shame, and then I may focus on the pain of this emotion and tell myself that I cannot bear this emotional pain (discomfort disturbance).

REBT's focus on meta-disturbance

REBT theorists recognize that once a person disturbs themself, it often happens that they then disturb themself about this original disturbance. This is known as *meta-disturbance* (literally disturbance about disturbance), and I gave an example of this at the end of the previous section. So, REBT has a decided focus on meta-disturbance. It also distinguishes between different types of meta-disturbance. Thus, it argues that a person can disturb themself about:

- Disturbed emotions at C. A person may disturb themself either because of the pain of the emotional experience (e.g. 'I cannot stand the pain of feeling depressed') or because of the meaning the disturbed emotion has for the person (e.g. 'Feeling depressed is a weakness and proves that I am a weak person').

- Dysfunctional behaviour or action tendencies at C. Here the person focuses on what they did or what they felt like doing but did not do, and disturbs themself about one or the other, primarily because of the meaning the behaviour or action tendency has for the person (e.g. 'I felt like punching her lights out, which is really nasty and proves that I am a nasty person').

- Distorted cognitions at C. Here a person may focus on a distorted cognition, which becomes their new A, and disturbs themself about the meaning that such a thought has for them. Thus, suppose the person disturbs themself about finding a young person attractive and thinks that they may abuse the person (their distorted cognitive consequence at C). They may then disturb themself about this thought because they infer that is shameful and that they are a disgusting person for having it.

REBT's position on the origin and maintenance of psychological problems

We have seen that one of the key theoretical principles of REBT is that summarized in the maxim: 'People are not disturbed by events but by the rigid and extreme attitudes that they hold towards these events.' This means that while adversities contribute to the development of psychological disturbance, mainly when these events are highly aversive, disturbance occurs when people bring their tendencies to hold rigid and extreme attitudes towards these events.

Most approaches to CBT are based on social learning principles, whereby it is held that people learn to disturb themselves. REBT theorists also argue that human disturbance is partly learned, but it is unique among the CBT approaches in claiming that the biological basis of human irrationality and related disturbance is often more influential than the social learning basis. Thus, in a seminal paper, Ellis (1976) put forward several arguments in favour of the 'biological hypothesis', as it is known in REBT circles. Here are a few of Ellis's arguments:

1. People easily transform their strong preferences into rigid demands and have a difficult time giving up these demands and sticking to their strong, flexible preferences.
2. People are rarely taught to procrastinate and live self-undisciplined lives, but millions do so.
3. People easily fall back into self-defeating patterns after they have made progress in dealing constructively with these patterns.

4. People can easily give other people sound advice on dealing with their problems, but find it difficult to apply this advice consistently to themselves when they experience the same problems.

REBT theorists do not, therefore, have an elaborate view on the origins of disturbance. Having said this, they do acknowledge that it is easy for humans when they are young to disturb themselves about highly aversive events. However, they argue that, even under these conditions, people react differently to the same event, and thus we need to understand what a person brings to and takes from an adversity. People learn their standards and goals from their culture, but disturbance occurs when they bring their rigid and extreme attitudes to circumstances where their standards are not met, and the pursuit of their goals is blocked.

By contrast, REBT theorists have a more elaborate view of how psychological disturbance is maintained. They argue that people perpetuate their disturbance for several reasons, including the following:

- They lack the insight that their psychological disturbance is underpinned by their rigid and extreme attitudes and think instead that events cause it.
- They think that once they understand that their problems are underpinned by rigid and extreme attitudes, this understanding alone will lead to change.
- They do not work persistently to change their rigid and extreme attitudes and to integrate the flexible and non-extreme alternatives to these attitudes into their attitudinal system.
- They continue to act in ways that are consistent with their rigid and extreme attitudes.
- They disturb themselves about their original disturbances.
- They lack or are deficient in critical social skills, communication skills, problem-solving skills and other life skills.
- They think that their disturbance has pay-offs that outweigh the advantages of the healthy alternatives to their disturbed feelings and/or behaviour.
- They live in environments which support the rigid and extreme attitudes that underpin their problems.

As will be seen in the next section, REBT's view on the perpetuation of psychological disturbance informs its position on psychological change

Choice-based constructivism and good mental health

REBT theorists favour what might be called choice-based constructivism in that REBT argues that humans have choices when their hold preferences (e.g. 'I want you to like me'). Thus, they can construct a rigid attitude from this preference ('I want you to like me...and, therefore, you must do so') or a flexible attitude from the same preference (e.g. 'I want you to like me... but you do not have to do so'). Although a person may have a biologically based tendency to construct a rigid attitude when their preference is strong, they do not have to do this and can choose to construct a flexible attitude instead. The extent to which the person does this in a meaningful way depends on the extent to which they are prepared to 'go against the grain' and think and act according to the less powerful flexible attitude preference and refrain from thinking and acting according to their more powerful rigid attitude.

REBT theorists have a clear position on what constitutes good mental health, with flexibility and non-extremeness at its heart. Here is a partial list of such criteria which is self-explanatory: personal responsibility; flexibility and anti-extremism; scientific thinking and non-utopian in outlook; enlightened self-interest; social interest; self-direction; high tolerance of uncertainty; strong commitment to meaningful pursuits; calculated risk-taking and long-range hedonism.

The distinctive practical features of REBT

In this section, I will consider REBT's major distinctive practical features. In order to put these features in context, I begin by outlining REBT's position on therapeutic change.

REBT's view of psychological change

REBT has a realistic view of psychological change and encourages clients to accept that change is hard work, and consequently it urges therapists to be forceful, energetic and persistent as long as doing so does not threaten the therapeutic alliance (Dryden & Neenan, 2004). It also encourages clients to understand and implement the REBT change process by:

- Realizing that they largely create their own psychological problems and that while situations contribute to these problems, they are in general of lesser importance in the change process.
- Fully recognizing that they can address and overcome these problems.
- Setting goals.
- Understanding that their problems stem largely from rigid and extreme attitudes and that adopting alternative flexible and non-extreme attitudes will help them to achieve their goals.
- Detecting their rigid and extreme attitudes and discriminating between them and their flexible and non-extreme attitudes.

- Examining their rigid and extreme attitudes and their flexible and non-extreme attitudes until they see clearly that the former are false, illogical and unconstructive, while the latter are true, sensible and constructive.
- Working towards the internalization of their new flexible and non-extreme attitudes by using a variety of cognitive (including imaginal), emotive and behavioural change methods. In particular, clients are advised to act in ways that are consistent with the flexible and non-extreme attitudes that they wish to develop and to refrain from acting in ways that are consistent with their old rigid and extreme attitudes.
- Identifying and dealing with obstacles to change.
- Implementing relapse prevention procedures.
- Generalizing change to other relevant situations.
- Accepting themselves for backsliding and continuing to use REBT change techniques.
- Extending this process of examining attitudes and using multimodal methods of change into other areas of their lives and committing to doing so for as long as necessary.

REBT's position on the importance of the therapeutic relationship

The therapeutic relationship in REBT is deemed to be important, but not curative, and draws fully on working alliance theory (Bordin, 1979) as a way of understanding the significance of bonds, views, goals and tasks in REBT (Dryden, 2009). In brief, effectiveness in REBT is enhanced when the therapist and the client:

- Have a well-*bond*ed relationship in which the client experiences the therapist as understanding both their feelings and the attitudes that underpin these feelings, as accepting them as fallible human beings and as genuine in the therapeutic encounter. In this respect, Ellis (in Dryden, 1997) cautioned REB therapists against being overly warm with clients so as not to reinforce the latters' needs for love and approval. In general, REB therapists consider that clients' experiences of these therapist-offered 'core conditions' (Rogers, 1957) are deemed to be important, but neither necessary nor sufficient for enduring client change (Ellis, 1959).
- Share common *views* on such matters as problem assessment, 'case'. formulation, treatment and practical issues concerning therapy.
- Share an agreed vision concerning client treatment *goals*.
- Understand one another's *tasks* concerning what needs to be done for client goals to be met and can commit to carrying out their respective tasks.

While REB therapists adopt an active-directive stance in therapy, particularly at its outset, they are not prescriptive about how to implement that stance in terms of therapeutic style. Thus, it is possible for REB therapists to be informal or formal, humorous or serious, self-disclosing or non-self-disclosing, Socratic or didactic, and use metaphors, parables and stories or refrain from their use. Skilful REB therapists vary their therapeutic style according to the client that they are working with and the stage of therapy that they have reached. Also, while REB therapists are mindful of the many ways in which their clients differ, they argue that each person is a unique individual and it would be wrong to make assumptions about a person because of their age, race, gender and cultural background, for example. Instead, REB therapists seek to modify the therapeutic relationship based on the person's unique preferences. A question I routinely ask clients is: 'For me to be most helpful, is there anything you feel it is important for me to know about your culture, ethnicity, religion, language, sexual orientation, gender identity/expression, mental or physical health, or another factor?'

REBT's position on case formulation

REB therapists take a flexible approach to case formulation, using this to guide interventions, particularly in complex cases. However, they argue that one can do good therapy without making such a formulation and hold that frequently this formulation can be developed during therapy rather than fully at its outset. However, when a 'case' is deemed to be complicated, or a client is not making expected progress, then doing a more formal and extensive case formulation may be indicated; see Dryden (1998) for a full discussion on the REBT approach to case formulation, which is outside the scope of this chapter.

REBT's psychoeducational emphasis

REBT has a decided psychoeducational emphasis, and its practitioners argue that its theory of disturbance and change, as well as its core concepts, can actively be taught to and learned and implemented by clients. This principle is underpinned by the idea that REB therapists are very explicit about the REBT model and actively teach it to clients at an early stage so that they can give their informed consent before proceeding with this form of therapy.

While REBT can be practised in many ways, its skills of assessing and addressing problems can be directly taught to clients so that they can learn to be their own therapists almost from the outset. Indeed, some of the materials that have been devised to help clients to learn REBT self-help skills can also be used by people who wish to help themselves without formal therapy (e.g. Dryden, 2001) In addition, there are a number of REBT self-help books based on particular themes that also serve the same purpose (e.g. Dryden, 1999).

Skilled REB therapists will work explicitly with clients so that together they can choose whether and when to take a skills-teaching and learning approach to REBT.

REBT's preferred treatment order

REBT recommends a preferred order of treatment and argues that client problems should ideally be dealt with in the following order: a) disturbance, b) dissatisfaction, and c) development. Disturbance is deemed to be present when the client is facing an adversity and holds a set of rigid and extreme attitudes towards that adversity. The resultant dysfunctional ways of responding (emotionally, behaviourally and cognitively) mean that the client is ill-equipped to deal with the adversity while they are in a disturbed frame of mind. When they deal successfully with their disturbance, they are then ready to deal with the dissatisfaction of facing the adversity since at this point the client holds a set of flexible and non-extreme attitudes towards the adversity which has now become a focus for dissatisfaction rather than disturbance. Development issues, as the name implies, concern the client exploring ways of developing themself so that they can get the most out of their potential. They will not be able to do this as effectively as they could, until they have dealt with the dissatisfaction of having an adversity in her life. Thus, their REB therapist would encourage them to take steps to change the adversity if it can be changed or adjust constructively to the adversity if it can't be changed – while holding flexible and non-extreme attitudes, rather than rigid and extreme attitudes – before focusing their attention on development issues, if the client is seeking help in this area. Such work might be better described as REB coaching rather than REB therapy

While this is the preferred REBT order and a clear rationale will be given to and discussed with the client for using this order, if the latter is adamant that they want to use a different order, then the therapist will be mindful of the working alliance (see above). As such, they will encourage the client to proceed according to their preferences and review the results of doing so at a later date. There is little to be gained and much to be lost by the therapist attempting to force a client to use the preferred REBT order when they are very reluctant to do so. Indeed, an REB therapist who does this is likely to hold rigid ideas about how REBT must be practised and is thus being unhelpfully dogmatic!

A second area where REBT has views on the order of treatment concerns whether to deal with meta-disturbance issues before disturbance issues or vice versa. The preferred order is to deal with a meta-disturbance issue first if a) its presence interferes with the client working on the disturbance issue in or out of the session, b) it is clinically the most critical issue of the two and centrally, from a working alliance perspective, c) the client sees the sense of doing so.

Reshaping rigid and extreme attitudes

As outlined in the theoretical section above, REBT theory hypothesizes that a client's rigid and extreme attitudes largely determine their psychological problems and, of the two, rigid attitudes are at the very core of such disturbance.

It follows from this that REB therapists target for change their clients' rigid and extreme attitudes, and particularly the former, as early in therapy as is feasible. Other approaches in the CBT tradition (see Wills, 2008) argue that to focus on such underlying attitudes early in therapy will engender resistance because people are deemed to be reluctant to make deep structure change in preference to surface structure change. REB therapists argue differently and hold that as long as clients understand the role that such rigid and extreme attitudes play in determining and maintaining their problems and appreciate that they need to examine and change these attitudes if they are to address their problems effectively, then such resistance is kept to a minimum. It is important, therefore, to realize that skilful REB therapists minimize resistance on this issue because the work that they are doing with their clients is based firmly on a strong working alliance between the two.

Perhaps the most distinctive feature about REBT practice is the effort that REB therapists make to help their clients change their rigid and extreme attitudes to flexible and non-extreme attitudes, once they have identified the former and helped their clients construct the latter. This process involves several steps.

The first step in helping clients to change their rigid and extreme attitudes to their flexible and non-extreme alternatives is to assist them in detecting the former. In the first instance, this involves teaching clients about these dysfunctional attitudes and their nature. They are characterized by rigidity and by being extreme. Rigid attitudes occur most frequently in the form of demands and musts, and extreme attitudes which are derived from these rigid attitudes take the form of awfulizing attitudes, unbearability attitudes and devaluation (of self, others and life conditions) attitudes. REB therapists use several ways to teach clients about this vital aspect of REBT theory and help them to apply this knowledge in the assessment process to detect the dysfunctional attitudes that underpin their emotional problems.

The second step to helping clients to examine and change their rigid and extreme attitudes is to encourage them to construct alternative flexible and non-extreme attitudes and to understand that holding these attitudes will help them to achieve their therapeutic goals.

As guided by REBT theory, if the therapist is targeting a rigid attitude for change (e.g. 'You must like me'), they first need to help the client to construct a flexible attitude (e.g. 'I want you to like me, but you do not have to do so'). Moreover, if the therapist is targeting an extreme attitude (i.e. an awfulizing attitude, an unbearability attitude or a devaluation attitude), they first need to help the client construct a non-extreme attitude (i.e. a non-awfulizing attitude, a bearability attitude or an unconditional acceptance attitude). Thus, if the therapist is targeting an extreme, awfulizing attitude (e.g. 'It would be awful if you don't like me'), they would first help the client to construct an alternative non-extreme, non-awfulizing attitude (e.g. 'It would be bad if you don't like me, but it would not be awful'). If the therapist fails to help the client to construct a flexible and/or non-extreme attitude alternative to their rigid and/or extreme attitude, then they will impede the change process as the client will be in an attitude vacuum, having been encouraged to give up their dysfunctional attitude, but without anything to replace it with.

The third step in helping clients to change their rigid and extreme attitudes to their flexible and non-extreme alternatives is encouraging them to differentiate their rigid and extreme attitudes from their constructed flexible and non-extreme attitudes. In the same way that REB therapists educate their clients to understand what dysfunctional attitudes are and the forms that they take, they also teach them to understand what functional attitudes are and the forms that they take.

A very important part of this process is helping clients to understand keenly the differences between dysfunctional and functional attitudes. For example, it is not sufficient to show a client that the functional alternative to their (in this case) rigid attitude 'I must impress my new boss straight-away' is the attitude 'I would like to impress my new boss straightaway'. The latter may not be rigid, but it is not fully flexible. While it asserts her preference, it does not negate her demand. The flexible alternative to her rigid attitude is: 'I would like to impress my new boss straightaway, but I do not have to do so', which incorporates both components of the flexible attitude. Table 1.1 outlines clearly the full differences between rigid and extreme attitudes, on the one hand, and flexible and non-extreme attitudes, on the other.

Examining clients' rigid and extreme attitudes and flexible and non-extreme attitudes

After REB therapists have helped their clients to see the differences between their dysfunctional and functional attitudes, they move on to help their clients to question or examine these attitudes. Albert Ellis (1994) referred to this process as 'disputing', which I call 'examining' here. This is done after clients understand the relationship between their rigid and extreme attitudes

Table 1.1 **Rigid/extreme and flexible/non-extreme attitudes in REBT theory**

Rigid and extreme attitude	Flexible and non-extreme attitude
Rigid attitude X must (or must not) happen 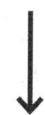	*Flexible attitude* I would like X to happen (or not happen), but it does not have to be the way I want it to be 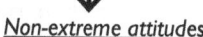
Extreme attitudes	*Non-extreme attitudes*
<u>Awfulizing attitude</u> It would be terrible if X happens (or does not happen)	<u>Non-awfulizing attitude</u> It would be bad, but not terrible if X happens (or does not happen)
<u>Unbearability attitude</u> I could not bear it if X happens (or does not happen)	<u>Bearability attitude</u> It would be difficult to bear if X happens (or does not happen), but I could bear it, it would be worth it to me to do so, I am willing to bear it and I am going to do so
<u>Devaluation attitude</u> If X happens (or does not happen), I am no good/you are no good/life is no good	<u>Unconditional acceptance attitude</u> If X happens (or does not happen), it does not prove that I am no good/ you are no good/life is no good. Rather, I am/you are a fallible human being and life is a complex mixture of good, bad and neutral

and their emotional problems and their flexible and non-extreme attitudes and their goals. What follows applies both to clients' specific attitudes and their more general attitudes.

As DiGiuseppe (1991) has shown, 'examining' involves questioning both clients' rigid and extreme attitudes and flexible and non-extreme attitudes to the point where they see the reasons for the dysfunctionality of the former (i.e. they are false, illogical and lead largely to poor results) and for the functionality of the latter (i.e. they are true, logical and lead largely to good results). Also, short didactic explanations are given until clients reach the same insight. These questions/explanations are directed to clients' rigid and flexible attitudes as well as to their extreme and non-extreme attitudes, and this is done using a variety of styles (see below).

In common with other CB therapists, REB therapists ask clients questions about the empirical status and the pragmatic status of their attitudes.

However, they also ask them about the logical status of their attitudes (e.g. 'Which is more logical, your attitude "Because I want to do well, therefore I have to" or the alternative attitude "I do not have to do well even though I want to"?'). Other CB therapists do this less frequently, and thus this is a distinctive feature of REBT. It may be that empirical ('Is it true?') and pragmatic arguments ('Is it helpful?') are more persuasive to clients than logical arguments ('Is it logical?'); we do not know because the relevant research has not been done. Even if this is the case, in general REB therapists would still use logical questioning/disputing of attitudes for two reasons. First, they do not know, on a priori grounds, which clients will find which arguments most persuasive in changing their rigid and extreme attitudes to their flexible and non-extreme alternatives. Just because the majority of clients may find logical arguments unpersuasive, it does not follow that all will do so and to withhold such arguments from those who might find them persuasive would not be good practice. So, REB therapists tend to use all three arguments to see, as I said above, which arguments will be most persuasive with which clients.

Second, REB therapists use empirical, pragmatic and logical arguments while questioning/disputing attitudes in order to cover all the bases (comprehensiveness). This comprehensiveness may itself be productive. Thus, even if clients find empirical and pragmatic arguments more persuasive than logical arguments, it may still be worthwhile employing such arguments in that they may add value to the overall effectiveness of the questioning/disputing process. Some clients may find it persuasive that their dysfunctional attitudes are false, unhealthy and illogical even if they find the logical argument weak on its own.

REBT recommends teaching general flexible and non-extreme philosophies to clients whenever feasible

While REB therapists will, as a matter of course, encourage their clients to acquire, develop and maintain specific flexible and non-extreme attitudes, they will also, whenever possible, offer to teach them general flexible and non-extreme philosophies and encourage them to make a 'profound philosophic change' – for example, changing general rigid attitudes, such as 'I must be liked by significant people', to general flexible attitudes, such as 'I want to be liked by significant people, but they do not have to like me', if they are capable of doing so and interested in doing so. Not all clients, will be so capable and/or interested, but if therapists do not offer to do this, they may be depriving a significant minority of their clients of getting the most out of REBT.

Compromises in REBT

REB therapists have a preferred strategy and, as we have seen, this involves encouraging clients to achieve attitude change. However, REBT recognizes that clients may not be able or willing to change their rigid and extreme attitudes and, in such cases, it recommends making compromises with the ideal of attitude change (Dryden, 1987a). Thus, when a client is not able or willing to change their dysfunctional attitudes, the REBT practitioner can help them to:

1. change their distorted inferences;
2. change their behaviour;
3. learn new skills;
4. change or leave the situation in which they experience their problem.

Change-based versus acceptance-based focus

One of the significant recent developments within the CBT tradition has been the growth of those CBT approaches which recommend that clients mindfully accept the presence of dysfunctional cognitions and troublesome feelings without engaging with them. This may be thought of as an acceptance-based focus and is typical of what has become known as 'third-wave CBT'. REBT (which would be regarded as a 'second-wave' CBT approach), on the other hand, generally recommends that clients identify, challenge and change rigid and extreme attitudes (at *B*) in the *ABC* framework, and respond, usually afterwards, to distorted inferences (either at *A* or at *C*). In short, REBT recommends that clients mindfully engage with troublesome cognitions (i.e. attitudes and inferences) to change them. This may be known as a change-based focus.

While it may be thought that these two foci cannot both be utilized in REBT, I believe they can. Here is how I make use of both a change-based focus, where attitudes and inferences are targeted for change, and an acceptance-based focus, where these cognitions are mindfully accepted.

- I use a change-based focus when encouraging clients to examine or question their rigid and extreme attitudes in the first instance. When clients consider that they have got as much out of this focus as they can on any particular occasion, I encourage them to shift to an acceptance-based focus if the dysfunctional attitudes are still in their mind. It is unrealistic to expect a person to be convinced fully of their change-based focus interventions in any single questioning episode.
- With highly distorted cognitive consequences of rigid and extreme attitudes, I initially teach clients to understand why these thoughts are so distorted (i.e. they are the product of dysfunctional attitudes). I then help them to use the presence of these thoughts to identify the rigid and extreme attitudes that have spawned them and then to use a change-based focus (CBF) with these dysfunctional attitudes. I may subsequently help them to use the same change-based focus to respond to these cognitive *C*s but to recognize that these thoughts may still

reverberate in their mind, at which point I encourage them to switch to an acceptance-based focus (ABF). Such reverberation is a natural process as the mind does not switch off from such thoughts just because CBF methods have been successfully used on any one occasion.

As third-wave CB therapists note (e.g. Hayes, Strosahl & Wilson, 2012), little productive change can be achieved when clients get enmeshed and entwined with their dysfunctional (i.e. rigid and extreme) attitudes and distorted inferences, and it is then when I advocate the use of an acceptance-based focus. However, from an REBT perspective, little can be gained by failing to encourage clients to respond constructively to these cognitions by employing a change-based focus when they can do so.

It should be noted that this is one REB therapist's perspective concerning when to encourage clients to respond to problematic attitudes and inferences and when to accept them mindfully. However, it shows that REBT practitioners are open to consider what newer CBT approaches can offer the theory and practice of REBT.

Responding to clients' doubts, reservations and objections to REBT

Like other therapists, REBT practitioners address client obstacles to change. However, since REB therapists endeavour to teach clients salient REBT concepts, it often transpires that such obstacles are rooted in clients' doubts and reservations about or objections to these concepts. It frequently transpires that their doubts are based on client misconceptions of these concepts. If the REB therapist does not elicit clients' doubts, then the clients will still have these doubts and be influenced by them, and they will thus resist making changes. However, as the therapist has not elicited their clients' doubts, they will not know why the clients are resisting change. For example, a client sometimes thinks that their rigid attitudes in the form of 'musts' are helpful in the sense that they are motivating and, without them, the client would not strive towards their goals. In this case, the REB therapist would help the client understand that it is their preference (common to both their rigid and flexible attitude) that is motivational, but when this preference is made rigid, it creates psychological disturbance, which does not happen when the preference is kept flexible.

Emphasis on therapeutic efficiency

All therapeutic approaches are (or should be) concerned with matters of therapeutic effectiveness. REBT is also concerned with the principle of therapeutic efficiency – bringing about change in the briefest time possible (Ellis, 1980). This is why Ellis counsels REB therapists to adopt an early focus on clients' rigid and extreme attitudes (see above) and to encourage their clients to tackle their problems full-on, if possible. Ellis's concern with therapeutic efficiency had its roots in his early experiences of carrying out lengthy diagnostic procedures with clients who dropped out before the treatment phase began, which he regarded as a waste of a clinician's time and thus therapeutically inefficient (Ellis, 1962).

REBT is an eclectic therapy

Although REBT is clearly placed in the tradition of CBT, it can also be regarded as an eclectic therapy. Indeed, I have called REBT a form of theoretically consistent eclecticism – advocating the broad use of techniques, from wherever, but to achieve goals in keeping with REBT theory (Dryden, 1987b). However, it sometimes will use techniques that are not in keeping with REBT theory when theoretically consistent techniques bear no therapeutic fruit (see Ellis, 2002). Thus, emotional freedom techniques (EFT) are not in keeping with REBT theory, but can be tried when all else fails (Craig, 2011). Ultimately, REB therapists' primary concern is to help their clients rather than to practise REBT!

Research on Rational Emotive Behaviour Therapy

There has been a considerable amount of research done on the relationship between irrational attitudes and psychological distress and the outcome of REBT. Space constraints mean that I will only refer to meta-analytic and other comprehensive reviews.

The relationship between rigid and extreme attitudes and psychological disturbance

Vîslă and colleagues (2016) reviewed the relationship between rigid and extreme attitudes and psychological disturbance by examining a hundred independent samples in 83 studies. The results showed that, overall, rigid and extreme attitudes were positively associated with various types of disturbance, such as general distress, anxiety, depression, anger and guilt (omnibus: r = 0.38). This relationship between rigid and extreme attitudes and disturbance was robust in that the association was found across different samples, measurements and study designs. A more focused review conducted by Gellatly and Beck (2016) on the relationship between catastrophic thinking (a cognitive construct very similar to REBT's concept of awfulizing) and a variety of psychological problems, including anxiety disorders, PTSD, pain and physical disability, among others, found that such thinking was a feature of these disorders. The authors suggest that what might be called catastrophic attitudes be regarded as a transdiagnostic phenomenon and 'be recognized as a clinically and scientifically useful global construct for understanding multiple disorders' (Gellatly & Beck, 2016: 446).

The effectiveness of REBT

There have been several meta-analyses of studies on the effectiveness of REBT with adults (Engels, Garnefski, & Diekstra, 1993; Lyons & Woods, 1991) and with children and adolescents (Gonzalez et al., 2004; Trip, Vernon, & McMahon, 2007). However, as can be seen, the most recent meta-analysis with adults was undertaken well over twenty years ago and the latest with children and adolescents was more than ten years ago. Most of these meta-analyses were flawed in that they included a relatively small number of studies and did not look at the mechanisms of change. A recent meta-analysis (David et al., 2017) corrected these flaws. These authors carried out a systematic search and identified 84 articles, out of which 68 provided data for between-group analysis and 39 for within-group analysis. They found a medium effect size of REBT compared to other interventions on outcomes ($d = 0.58$) and on irrational attitudes ($d = 0.70$), at post-test. For the within-group analysis, they obtained medium effects for both outcomes ($d = 0.56$) and irrational attitudes ($d = 0.61$).

While changing rigid and extreme attitudes is a distinct feature of REBT, it should be noted that these attitudes can be changed by other CBT approaches, and REBT can change other forms of dysfunctional thinking (Cristea et al., 2015; Szentágotai, David, Lupu, & Cosman, 2008). As such, we do not have evidence that shows that REBT brings about change by restructuring clients' rigid and extreme attitudes rather than other forms of dysfunctional thinking, or that other CBT approaches do not change rigid and extreme attitudes.

Dissemination of REBT

Ellis and other REB therapists have been active over the years disseminating REBT ideas to both professional and public audiences.

Professional dissemination

When Ellis first developed REBT in the 1950s, he sent reel-to-reel tapes of his clinical work to therapists interested in finding out about REBT. He would take every opportunity to give talks on REBT and to write articles and chapters giving the REBT slant on whatever clinical issue was piquing people's interest as well as a steady stream of books showing how to practise REBT with a range of clinical disorders and populations. Also, other

REB therapists have written books on how to practise REBT with specific problems/populations and more generally. A notable example of the latter is the third edition of *A Practitioner's Guide to Rational Emotive Behaviour Therapy* (DiGiuseppe, Doyle, Dryden, & Backx, 2014).

In addition, what is now known as the Albert Ellis Institute has run a range of professional training courses in New York for many years, and its affiliated training centres throughout the world continue this tradition. However, studies evaluating these professional dissemination activities are still awaited.

Public dissemination

Ellis's (1957a) first book on REBT was written for the public, and throughout his long career he continued this tradition, authoring many self-help books on general and more focused issues. Other REB therapists who have continued this tradition include Paul Hauck and myself.

Ellis also pioneered what he called the 'Friday Night Workshop', an event for the public where Ellis would demonstrate REBT with two volunteers in front of a mainly lay audience. This has always proved a popular and vivid way of disseminating REBT principles to the public, which is helpful to both the volunteers themselves and the watching audience (Ellis & Joffe, 2002). The Albert Ellis Institute has continued to host this event, now known as 'Friday Night Live'.

These professional and public activities show that REBT is alive and that Ellis's wish for REBT principles to continue to be promulgated after his death is being fulfilled.

Conclusion

REBT is the oldest of the cognitive-behaviour therapies. Perhaps partly because of this, it struggles for professional attention in a therapeutic world where the novel is often more appealing than the traditional. However, it also seems to be the case that the theory and practice are not fully understood (see Dryden, 2013) and thus, in this chapter, I have placed much emphasis on outlining and discussing REBT's distinctive theoretical and practical distinctive features. For if a therapeutic approach is to be appropriately evaluated, it first needs to be properly understood!

Notes

1 In this chapter, I will use the term 'attitudes' rather than 'beliefs' since this term more accurately refers to the evaluative cognitions that are deemed to mediate between an adversity and a person's response to that adversity in REBT theory;

see Dryden (2016) for a detailed discussion of this point. To preserve the *B* in the *ABC* framework (see later), I use the term 'basic attitudes'.

2   Much of what appears in this section can be found in Ellis (2004).

References

Adler, A. (1927). *Understanding human nature*. New York: Garden City.

Adler, A. (1964). *Social interest: A challenge to mankind*. New York: Capricorn.

Bordin, E.S. (1979). The generalizability of the psychoanalytic concept of the working alliance. *Psychotherapy: Theory, Research and Practice, 16*, 252–260.

Bourland, Jr., D.D. (1965/1966). A linguistic note: Writing in e-prime. *General Semantics Bulletin, 32–33*, 111–114.

Craig, C. (2011). *The EFT manual*. Santa Rosa, CA: Energy Psychology Press.

Cristea, I.A., Huibers, M.J., David, D., Hollon, S.D., Andersson, G., & Cuijpers, P. (2015). The effects of cognitive behavior therapy for adult depression on dysfunctional thinking: A meta-analysis. *Clinical Psychology Review, 42*, 62–71.

David, D., Cotet, C., Matu, S., Magoase, C., & Stefan, S. (2017). 50 years of rational-emotive and cognitive-behavioral therapy: A systematic review and meta-analysis. *Journal of Clinical Psychology*. DOI: 10.1002/jclp.22514

DiGiuseppe, R. (1991). Comprehensive cognitive disputing in rational-emotive therapy. In M. Bernard (Ed.), *Using rational-emotive therapy effectively* (pp. 173–195). New York: Plenum.

DiGiuseppe, R.A., Doyle, K.A., Dryden, W., & Backx, W. (2014). *A practitioner's guide to rational emotive behaviour therapy. 3rd edition*. New York: Oxford University Press.

Dryden, W. (1987a). *Current issues in rational-emotive therapy*. London: Croom Helm.

Dryden, W. (1987b). A case of theoretically consistent eclecticism: Humanizing a computer "addict." In J.C. Norcross (Ed.), *Casebook of eclectic psychotherapy* (pp. 221–237). New York: Brunner/Mazel.

Dryden, W. (1997). *Therapists' dilemmas. Revised edition*. London: Sage.

Dryden, W. (1998). Understanding persons in the context of their problems: Rational emotive behaviour therapy perspective. In M. Bruch & F.W. Bond (Eds.), *Beyond diagnosis: Case formulation approaches in CBT* (pp. 43–64). Chichester: John Wiley & Sons.

Dryden, W. (1999). *How to accept yourself*. London: Sheldon Press.

Dryden, W. (2001). *Reason to change: A rational emotive behaviour therapy (REBT) workbook*. Hove, East Sussex: Brunner-Routledge.

Dryden, W. (2009). *Skills in rational emotive behaviour counselling and psychotherapy*. London: Sage.

Dryden, W. (2013). *The ABCs of REBT: Perspectives on conceptualization*. New York: Springer.

Dryden, W. (2015). *Rational emotive behaviour therapy: Distinctive features. 2nd edition*. Hove, East Sussex: Routledge.

Dryden, W. (2016). *Attitudes in rational emotive behaviour therapy: Components, characteristics and adversity-related consequences*. London: Rationality Publications.

Dryden, W., & Ellis, A. (1986). Rational-emotive therapy. In W. Dryden & W.L. Golden (Eds.), *Cognitive-behavioural approaches to psychotherapy* (pp. 129–168). London: Harper & Row.

Dryden, W., Ferguson, J., & McTeague, S. (1989). Attitudes and inferences: A test of a rational-emotive hypothesis. 2: On the prospect of seeing a spider. *Psychological Reports, 64*, 115–123.

Dryden, W., & Neenan, M. (2004). *The rational emotive behavioural approach to therapeutic change*. London: Sage Publications.

Ellis, A. (1955). New approaches to psychotherapy techniques. *Journal of Clinical Psychology Monograph Supplement, 11*, 1–53.

Ellis, A. (1957a). *How to live with a neurotic*. New York: Crown Publishers.

Ellis, A. (1957b). Rational psychotherapy and individual psychology. *Journal of Individual Psychology, 13*(1), 38–44.

Ellis, A. (1959). Requisite conditions for basic personality change. *Journal of Consulting Psychology, 23*, 538–540.

Ellis, A. (1962). *Reason and emotion in psychotherapy*. Secaucus, NJ: Lyle Stuart.

Ellis, A. (1973). *Humanistic psychotherapy: The rational-emotive approach*. New York: McGraw-Hill.

Ellis, A. (1976). The biological basis of human irrationality. *Journal of Individual Psychology, 32*, 145–168.

Ellis, A. (1980). The value of efficiency in psychotherapy. *Psychotherapy: Theory, Research and Practice, 17*, 414–419.

Ellis, A. (1981). The place of Immanuel Kant in cognitive psychotherapy. *Rational Living, 16*, 13–16.

Ellis, A. (1984). The essence of RET. *Journal of Rational-Emotive Therapy, 2*(1), 19–25.

Ellis, A. (1993). Changing rational-emotive therapy (RET) to rational emotive behavior therapy (REBT). *Behavior Therapist, 16*, 257–258.

Ellis, A. (1994). *Reason and emotion in psychotherapy. Revised and updated edition*. Secaucus, NJ: Carol.

Ellis, A. (1997). The evolution of Albert Ellis and rational emotive behavior therapy. In J.K. Zeig (Ed.), *The evolution of psychotherapy: The third conference* (pp. 69–82). New York: Brunner/Mazel.

Ellis, A. (1999). Why rational-emotive therapy to rational emotive behavior therapy. *Psychotherapy: Theory, Research and Practice, 36*, 154–159.

Ellis, A. (2002). *Overcoming resistance: A rational emotive behavior therapy integrated approach*. New York: Springer.

Ellis, A. (2004). *Rational emotive behavior therapy: It works for me – it can work for you*. Amherst, NY: Prometheus.

Ellis, A., & Harper, R.A. (1975). *A new guide to rational living*. North Hollywood, CA: Wilshire.

Ellis, A., & Joffe, D. (2002). A study of volunteer clients who experience live sessions of REBT in front of a public audience. *Journal of Rational-Emotive and Cognitive Behavior Therapy, 20*, 151–158.

Engels, G.I., Garnefski, N., & Diekstra, R.F. (1993). Efficacy of rational-emotive therapy: A quantitative analysis. *Journal of Consulting and Clinical Psychology, 61*, 1083–1090.

Gellatly, R., & Beck, A.T. (2016). Catastrophic thinking: A transdiagnostic process across psychiatric disorders. *Cognitive Therapy and Research, 40*, 1–12.

Gonzalez, J.E., Nelson, J.R., Gutkin, T.B., Saunders, A., Galloway, A., & Shwery, C.S. (2004). Rational-emotive therapy with children and adolescents: A meta-analysis. *Journal of Emotional and Behavioral Disorders, 12*, 222–235.

Hayes, S.C., Strosahl, K.D., & Wilson, K.G. (2012). *Acceptance and commitment therapy: The process and practice of mindful change. 2nd edition.* New York: Guilford.

Heidegger, M. (1949). *Existence and being.* Chicago, IL: Henry Regnery.

Hjelle, L.A., & Ziegler, D.J. (1992). *Personality theories: Basic assumptions, research and applications.* New York: McGraw-Hill.

Horney, K. (1950). *Neurosis and human growth.* New York: Norton.

Korzybski, A. (1933). *Science and sanity.* San Francisco, CA: International Society of General Semantics.

Lyons, L.C., & Woods, P.J. (1991). The efficacy of rational-emotive therapy: A quantitative review of the outcome research. *Clinical Psychology Review, 11*, 357–369.

Popper, K.R. (1959). *The logic of scientific discovery.* New York: Harper & Brothers.

Popper, K.R. (1963). *Conjectures and refutations.* New York: Harper & Brothers.

Reichenbach, H. (1953). *The rise of scientific philosophy.* Berkeley: University of California Press.

Rogers, C.R. (1957). The necessary and sufficient conditions of therapeutic personality change. *Journal of Consulting Psychology, 21*, 95–103.

Russell, B. (1930). *The conquest of happiness.* New York: New American Library.

Russell, B. (1965). *The basic writings of Bertrand Russell.* New York: Simon & Schuster.

Szentágotai, A., David, D., Lupu, V., & Cosman, D. (2008). Rational emotive behavior therapy versus cognitive therapy versus pharmacotherapy in the treatment of major depressive disorder: Mechanisms of change analysis. *Psychotherapy: Theory, Research, Practice, Training, 45*, 523–538.

Tillich, P. (1953). *The courage to be.* New Haven, CT: Yale University Press.

Trip, S., Vernon, A., & McMahon, J. (2007). Effectiveness of rational-emotive education: A quantitative meta-analytical study. *Journal of Cognitive and Behavioral Psychotherapies, 7*(1), 81–93.

Vîslă, A., Flückiger, C., grosse Holtforth, M.G., & David, D. (2016). Irrational beliefs and psychological distress: A meta-analysis. *Psychotherapy and Psychosomatics, 85*, 8–15.

Wills, F. (2008). *Skills in cognitive behaviour counselling and psychotherapy.* London: Sage Publications.

Ziegler, D.J. (2000). Basic assumptions concerning human nature underlying rational emotive behavior therapy (REBT) personality theory. *Journal of Rational-Emotive and Cognitive-Behavior Therapy, 18*, 67–85.

Chapter 2

REBT's place in modern psychotherapy[1]

Similarities with all psychotherapies, with other forms of CBT, and unique characteristics

Raymond DiGiuseppe

This chapter identifies REBT's position in modern psychotherapy. It identifies the characteristics that REBT shares with most other psychotherapies, such as the common factors model, psychodynamic therapies, and client-centered therapy. It explores the ideas, strategies, and techniques REBT shares with other treatments within the CBT psychotherapy tradition. It identifies REBT characteristics that have been adopted by other forms of CBT, such as Acceptance and Commitment Therapy, Cognitive Therapy, and Dialectical Behavior Therapy. Finally, the unique features of REBT are identified.

I often ask myself why I have remained an REBT (Rational Emotive Behavior Therapy) advocate for so long. I became affiliated with REBT when my dissertation mentor, Howard Kassinove, introduced me to the theory in 1973. I started a postdoctoral fellowship at the Albert Ellis Institute in 1975, and I have remained there ever since. Other theories have appeared during this period, and I have explored them but remain committed to REBT. This chapter results from my reflections on this question. I attempt to define REBT's place in psychotherapy in the early 21st century by exploring three questions. How is REBT like all psychotherapies? How does REBT compare with other forms of Cognitive Behavior Therapy (CBT), which are REBT's closest cousins? What are the unique features of REBT? Dryden (e.g., 2015) first outlined REBT's distinctive features, many of which have been adopted by other CBT schools and might now be common characteristics of CBT.

Aspects of REBT that are similar to all psychotherapies

REBT utilizes the common factors of psychotherapy

REBT includes many postulates and practices that are common to other accepted forms of psychotherapy. Presently research proposes that all

DOI: 10.4324/9781003081593-3

major psychotherapies are equally effective (a position with which I do not concur), and common factors contribute a significant amount of the variance in any psychotherapy's effectiveness (Wampold and Imel, 2015). This idea has a long history and was proposed first by Rosenzweig (1936) and later by Frank and Frank (1962). Ellis (1964) also recognized that common factors contribute to psychotherapy's effectiveness. These common factors include the following. Psychotherapy occurs in an emotionally charged and confiding relationship with a healer. Therapy takes place in a healing setting. The patient actively participates in the activities. The patient has positive expectations for change. Wampold and Imel (2015) identified some additional features of the common factors model. These include the following: (1) the development of the therapeutic alliance, which includes agreement on the goals and tasks of therapy and the formation of a therapeutic bond, (2) the patient accepts an explanation of their problems offered by the psychotherapist, and (3) the patient agrees with a rationale for the treatment that is consistent with the rationale of the client's problems, (4) the psychotherapist's allegiance to a theory positively influences the outcome, and (5) the psychotherapist's adherence to the therapy model is not associated with the outcome. Ellis and most REBT practitioners would agree with all of these aspects of the common activities except the statement on the role of adherence. REBT's psychoeducational nature ensures that practitioners provide patients with a rationale for their disturbance and the treatment (Ellis, 1962). By teaching patients the A-B-C model that explains the relationship between irrational beliefs (IBs) and disturbance, REBT practitioners are likely to develop agreement on psychotherapy tasks.

The crucial aspects of the therapeutic alliance are reaching an agreement on the goals and tasks of psychotherapy. Having listened to hundreds of Ellis's sessions, I observed Ellis routinely reaching agreement on his patients' therapeutic goals and the session's long-term and immediate goals. Ellis began his session by asking the client to identify issues they wanted to discuss in the current session. Also, Ellis explained the process of therapy to his patients and sought their agreement. The importance of attaining agreement on therapy goals and tasks is still stressed today (DiGiuseppe et al., 2014). These strengths of REBT emphasize the elements that Frank and Frank (1962) and Wampold and Imel (2015) see as common factors of psychotherapy. Perhaps Ellis, consciously or unconsciously, was influenced by the Franks' work and infused these aspects of the common factors model into REBT.

Features that REBT shares with psychodynamic therapy

Psychodynamic therapy (PD) has had a significant and lasting effect on psychotherapy. The primary mechanism of change in PD is the analysis of the transference. Through discussions about the patient's interactions with the psychotherapist, the patient becomes aware of the conflicts they typically have with significant others. The therapy makes these unconscious conflicts conscious. REBT differs from PD in that REBT does not identify the transference analysis as an essential mechanism for change, although it might contribute to change. REBT is much more active than PD. REBT is psychoeducational and teaches patients to challenge what they think and develop new ways of thinking.

Because Ellis initially practiced PD, many aspects of PD are likely to appear in REBT. Shedler (2010) identified seven distinctive features of PD, and an examination of Shedler's distinctive features illuminates some similarities between REBT and this dominant form of psychotherapy.

1. *Focusing on emotions.* Shedler (2010) notes that PD focuses on affect and the expression of emotion. PD encourages exploration and discussion of the full range of a patient's emotions. The therapist helps the patient describe the feelings that are threatening and identifies feelings patients might not recognize. REBT does this. Shedler says that CBTs place greater emphasis on thoughts and beliefs. Without understanding the patient's emotions, REBT and CBT practitioners could not identify the appropriate IBs. REBT has a more complex theory of emotions than most psychotherapies and, as such, stresses emotions in a manner not acknowledged by PD theorists.
2. *Exploring the avoidance of distressing thoughts and emotions.* PD posits that most symptoms are knowingly and unknowingly attempts to avoid uncomfortable experiences. PD therapists actively explore such avoidances. This principle of PD represents REBT's focus on meta or secondary disturbance, which Dryden (2015) identified as a distinctive feature of REBT. Such avoidance is also a key element of Acceptance and Commitment Therapy (ACT) and Dialectical Behavior Therapy (DBT: Matweychuk et al., 2019). Perhaps Ellis developed his position on secondary disturbance from his PD training. However, REBT, as well as ACT and DBT, do not rely on the analysis of the transference or insight to change secondary disturbance but use more active behavioral and cognitive strategies to do so.
3. *Identifying recurring themes.* PD psychotherapists explore recurring themes and patterns in patients' thoughts, feelings, self-concept, and relationships. Problems that patients present are often an example of a theme that permeates their life. Competent psychotherapists observe such patterns, which inform the therapist about the significant issues (and IBs) in the patient's life that can be targeted for change. This distinctive feature of PD is consistent with REBT and seems more to be a common psychotherapy factor.
4. *Discussion of past experience (a developmental focus).* Related to identifying recurring themes and patterns, PD postulates that early

experiences with attachment figures affect people's present relationships. PD psychotherapists explore early experiences because they believe that the past "lives on" in the present. REBT is more present-focused than PD. REBT acknowledges that it could help to explore the patient's history to understand and change their present problems. REBT posits that people might have learned their IBs from their family, peers, or society. However, it is rehearsing these thoughts that is the most critical factor leading to disturbance. Also, REBT posits that people can construct their IBs without input from others. Also, REBT advocates that people take responsibility for their disturbing emotions and change their IBs. Would REBT practitioners sometimes explore the past? Ellis once attributed to Freud an idea that the past is important because people continue to carry it around with them. Ellis then added that people indoctrinate themselves in their past IBs. The importance of focusing on the past is a clear difference between REBT and PD. REBT puts less emphasis on exploring the past than would PD.

5. *Focusing on interpersonal relations.* PD places heavy emphasis on patients' relationships and interpersonal experience. PD psychotherapists explore how the patient experiences their interpersonal relations. Ellis (1962) noted that humans are social, and it is in a person's best interest to get along with others, as this will lead to less disturbance and positive adjustment. Thus, this distinctive feature does not seem unique to PD. REBT stresses the same focus. Focusing on interpersonal relationships might be a common characteristic of effective psychotherapy.

6. *Focusing on the therapeutic relationship.* For PD, the recurrence of interpersonal themes in the therapy relationship (transference and countertransference) provides an opportunity to improve those relationships. PD strives to have the patient achieve greater flexibility in interpersonal relationships and enhance their satisfaction with relationships. This goal is primarily accomplished by analyzing the transference and focusing on the patient's relationship with the psychotherapist. The type of and purpose of the patient–therapist relationship is quite different in PD and REBT. Although REBT strives to accomplish a good therapeutic alliance as discussed above, analysis of the transference is not encouraged. Countertransference, the therapist's attitudes and emotions towards the patient, can bias their perceptions and interfere with treatment. This topic is often discussed in REBT (Ellis, 2002) and is frequently encountered and addressed in REBT supervision (Beal & DiGiuseppe, 1998).

7. *Exploring fantasy life.* Shedler (2010) maintains that PD encourages patients to speak freely about whatever is on their minds. Explorations of what patients fear might happen or what they want to happen are essential information to understand a patient and for setting treatment

goals. REBT would encourage such exploration as well. We know that people have fantasies concerning awfulizing events they imagine and desires that they believe are inappropriate and condemnable. This distinctive feature of PD is often practiced in REBT.

REBT shares many characteristics with PD. However, most of these shared characteristics involve identifying essential issues that help the psychotherapist understand the client. PD believes that insight and awareness are sufficient for change, and the analysis of transference is the best method to achieve this insight. REBT sees insight as the first step. Once a patient knows what issue they are upset about, they could change but most likely would need to challenge their IBs about that issue and learn to adopt RBs (rational beliefs).

Psychotherapists' effects on outcome

Wampold and Imel (2015) report that considerable variance in psychotherapy outcome is attributed to the person of the therapist. Psychotherapists matter and some individual traits and behaviors discriminate between the most effective psychotherapists and average or less effective ones. This idea is not foreign to REBT. Among a sample of therapists trained in REBT at the AEI (Albert Ellis Institute), the percentage of variance on outcome measures attributed to the psychotherapists is similar to that found in other studies where the therapists follow different therapies (Radosevich, 2009). Ellis regularly lectured on the characteristics of effective REB therapists (see Woods & Ellis, 1996). Ellis's list of attributes of effective psychotherapists and Wampold and Imel's (2015) list of empirically supported characteristics are remarkably similar. Both lists identify effective psychotherapists as possessing verbal fluency, having good interpersonal perception, modulating their emotions effectively, expressing warmth towards patients, offering unconditional acceptance towards patients, and having empathy.

The common factors model and REBT posit the same psychotherapists' characteristics of effective psychotherapists. Competent psychotherapists have sophisticated interpersonal skills. Clients of effective therapists feel understood. Effective therapists can form a working alliance with a broad range of clients. Effective psychotherapists provide an acceptable and adaptive explanation for the client's distress. The effective therapist is influential, persuasive, and convincing. They present an explanation for the patient's problems and the rationale for the treatment plan convincingly to the client. For REBT, we would go further and say the therapist is convincing and persuasive in challenging IBs and supporting RBs. The competent therapist continually monitors the client's progress. Effective therapists are flexible and can adjust therapy if resistance to the treatment is apparent or the client is not making progress. Effective psychotherapists do not avoid difficult material in therapy. They communicate hope and optimism and are aware of their psychological process. Competent therapists seek to improve continually.

Ellis added one characteristic not appearing on Wampold and Imel's list: competent therapists are highly intelligent.

The psychotherapy relationship

Although REBT's interventions naturally lead to two aspects of the therapeutic alliance, agreement on both the goals and the tasks of psychotherapy, we have not yet discussed the alliance's third aspect, the therapeutic bond. REBT has long been criticized as being too harsh and failing to develop good relationships with clients, and not fostering an authentic, warm relationship between psychotherapists and clients. DiGiuseppe et al. (1993) showed that REB therapists were rated by their patients as having relationship scores that were equal to or higher than any scores appearing in the literature when measuring the therapeutic relationship as defined by Rogers (1957). How did REBT develop the reputation of not building strong bonds between therapists and clients, and does it differ so much from other therapies on this dimension? Several factors might have contributed to this perception.

The Rogers–Ellis debate

In 1957, Ellis and Rogers debated the role of the therapeutic relationship. Rogers (1957) proposed that unconditional positive regard (UPR) by the psychotherapist for the client was a *necessary* and *sufficient* condition for human change. Ellis (1959) disagreed; he retorted that there are no necessary and sufficient conditions for human change. UPR was a highly desirable part of the therapeutic relationship and enormously facilitated change. However, it was not sufficient for change because many clients failed to improve despite receiving UPR from their therapists. UPR was not necessary for change because many people improved by other means without experiencing a psychotherapist's UPR. Although Ellis agreed that UPR was desirable and practiced it for decades in REBT (DiGiuseppe et al., 2014), many people remembered him for disagreeing with Rogers on the centrality of UPR.

Barber's hypothesis on the therapeutic relationship

Jacques Barber (2016) proposed an interesting historical reason that REBT and CBT are often perceived as not encouraging the therapeutic relationship. Ellis and Beck, the founders of REBT and Cognitive Therapy, received psychodynamic training that focused on the therapeutic bond (Hollon &

DiGiuseppe, 2011), and likely integrated these therapeutic relationship skills into their work with their new therapies; however, they failed to write about it. They wrote primarily on the difference between their unique approaches and the older ones. The second generation of CBT practitioners (e.g., J. Beck, DiGiuseppe, Dryden, Freeman, and Young) learned to integrate these relationship skills with the novel unique aspect of CBT by modeling their mentors.

The third generation of REBT and CBT practitioners never "learned" these skills because they neither appeared in books, nor were they discussed in workshops. Thus, the skills atrophied. Presently, the therapeutic relationship's importance is routinely taught in REBT and CBT, and research supports the idea these therapies are more effective when the psychotherapists have relationship-building skills (Castonguay et al., 2004). Ellis was very perceptive of his clients' emotions and problems, and he had an unusual ability to focus on their problems. He gave patients not only UPR but his intense sustained attention. You knew he was with you.

Ellis' distinction between feeling better and getting better

For decades, REBT has warned of the dilemma of expressing too much warmth towards clients (Ellis & Dryden, 1985). However, this does not translate into not expressing any warmth. Providing clients too much warmth might help them feel better without teaching them the skills to change their demands for love, which will help them get better. When Ellis was practicing PD, he noticed that many of his clients appear to improve because he had expressed warmth towards them (Ellis, 2002). As long as he was warm and loving towards them, they felt better. If he challenged their demands for his and other people's love, they would experience more discomfort. Ellis recognized that a psychotherapist could get short-term improvement in their clients by being warm; this also resulted in their staying in therapy longer and was financially advantageous to the therapist. However, such actions interfered with doing the hard work of challenging their IBs. Thus, they felt better without learning the skills to feel better if they did not experience warmth. Working on the clients' beliefs that they must be accepted required much more work and short-term discomfort, but produced more long-term benefits in terms of being less dependent on the therapist or anyone else. Thus, it might be in the patient's long-term interest to not be so warm, not develop a dependency on their psychotherapist, and learn to cope with not being loved.

Confrontation

Another reason for this perception is that Ellis frequently spoke about the importance of forcefully disputing patients' IBs. Some critics perceived this forceful disputing as confrontation. Confrontation in psychotherapy has two meanings. The first involves the psychotherapist pointing out inconsistencies or contradictions in the patient's behaviors, feelings, or thoughts. Reflecting on these inconsistencies helps patients develop insight concerning their genuine emotional reactions. The second definition refers to challenging the patient in a harsh, forceful manner. The second type of confrontation is often recommended in substance abuse treatment to have clients accept their drug use's destructive nature. All forms of psychotherapy use confrontation in the sense of the first definition. Using the second definition of confrontation, Ellis often advised therapists to be persistent and forceful in disputing patients' IBs (Ellis, 2002). However, Ellis's persistent and forceful disputing did not rise to the level of confrontation. Sometimes Ellis did dispute patients' IBs with a harsh confronting style. He would loudly raise his voice and challenge the patients to surrender their IBs and accept more rational alternatives.

Ellis' confrontive style was premeditated with patients who had not responded to traditional REBT or therapeutic styles. Ellis reported that since everything else he had tried with the patient had not worked, he attempted to shake them up and try something different. We have no evidence concerning whether Ellis's use of confrontation worked. Unfortunately, some REBT practitioners and trainers mimic this confrontive style when challenging patients' IBs and reinforce the idea that REBT requires a harsh challenging of the patients' IBs. Meta-analytic studies on the role of psychotherapists' behaviors on therapy outcomes conclude that harsh confrontation is negatively related to psychotherapy effectiveness (Norcross & Lambert, 2019). Consistent with this finding, most REBT practitioners and trainers do not use, teach, or model a harsh, confronting style when disputing patients' IBs (DiGiuseppe et al., 2014).

Comparisons of REBT with other Cognitive Behavior Therapies

The term Cognitive Behavior Therapy (CBT) was first used at a conference funded and hosted by the Albert Ellis Institute in 1977 (Hollon & DiGiuseppe, 2011). The main speakers were Al Ellis, Aaron Beck, Donald Meichenbaum, Michael Mahoney, and George Spivack to name a few. CBT represents an umbrella term that incorporates a broad therapeutic tradition of therapies. REBT has always been part of the CBT tradition that shares many features (Matweychuk et al., 2019). These similarities include: (1) employing relationship-building interventions, such as empathy, validation, and reflection, (2) identifying specific goals for therapy and sessions, (3) providing a theoretical explanation for the nature of patients' symptoms and an explanation for how the treatment works, (4) teaching behavioral skills and adaptive beliefs, (5) using experiential learning, (6) using summary statements within the session, (7) using activities such as exposure to fear and anger-provoking stimuli, behavioral activation, role-playing, and the modeling of adaptive behavior, (8) teaching problem-solving strategies, (9) using between-session homework to rehearse new behaviors and attitudes. However, most CBT models advocate questioning and evaluating dysfunctional thoughts and attitudes based on practical and empirical grounds and replacing them with more adaptive ideas. ACT advocates using only practical arguments aimed at the dysfunctional thoughts and not trying to replace them. Instead, this model advocates that patients learn to act more flexibly and act in accordance with their goals and values.

REBT has introduced many activities into the CBT tradition, which I will discuss below. In years past, we would have categorized many of the concepts as a unique characteristic of REBT. However, over time, REBT's distinctive features have gained acceptance and are now standard features of CBT.

Role of meta-disturbance

Ellis was one of the first theorists within the CBT tradition to identify that humans can disturb themselves about their internal experience. At point C, in the ABC model, people's emotions become an activating event that triggers irrational beliefs that lead to additional emotional arousal (Ellis 1980). Dryden (2015) identified this concept as "meta-disturbance" and as a distinctive feature of REBT. Thus, people can become depressed about their anxiety or anxious about their IBs. REBT advocates that psychotherapists target such meta-disturbance first, because the activation of these meta-disturbance beliefs interferes with all other interventions.

Shedler (2010) identified patients' avoidance of emotions because they were too painful to be experienced as a distinctive feature of PD. Several CBT models, such as ACT, DBT, Leahy's Emotional Schema Therapy (Leahy, 2018), and Wells' (2009) Meta-Cognitive Therapy stress the role that subjective experiences play in triggering emotional and behavioral disturbance and, like REBT, attempt to target these problems first. Although the role of meta-disturbance in psychopathology is a distinctive feature of REBT, it has been incorporated in many other therapies and is not unique to REBT. Meta-disturbance might be a common CBT feature or a transtheoretical concept.

The dual nature of human thoughts and emotions

Many models of psychotherapy acknowledge that humans have two parallel cognitive systems for processing information. Ellis always proposed that humans have the potential to think both rationally and irrationally. This idea was first proposed by the Dutch philosopher Spinoza, who suggested that people always have disturbing thoughts and that people learn new, more adaptive thoughts to counteract them (see Damasio, 2003). This idea is the central tenet of Daniel Kahneman's Nobel prize-winning theory outlined in his book *Thinking Fast and Thinking Slow* (2011). Kahneman contends that humans have a quick, irrational processing system that excites our alarm emotions and prepares us to react to threats. Although this system appears necessary for survival, it triggers many false positives. Humans have a second, slower, and more rational cognitive system that can override our fast reactions. Therapy tries to decrease the activation of our quick cognitive processing system and increase the engagement of our slow processing system. People can never eliminate the fast, irrational system; it is part of human nature. We can increase the speed and strength of the slow cognitive processing system to neutralize the fast system. Humans can learn the skill of challenging our irrationality whenever it might flare. Although REBT puts a strong emphasis on this dual processing model, most CBT models have incorporated this Ellis–Kahneman model.

Role of controlling thoughts

All CBT models are opposed to attempts to directly "control" thoughts. That is, CBT does not advocate for people not to have thoughts. There seems to be agreement that we cannot will thoughts away. Each therapy teaches clients some form of reaction to dysfunctional thoughts such as disputing, challenging, or restructuring the thoughts. CT and DBT attempt to test the veracity of negative thoughts, and ACT, skeptical of disputation strategies, avoids them and relies on functional arguments that dysfunctional thoughts do not help one accomplish goals.

Identification of alternative adaptive cognitions, emotions, and behaviors

All CBT models include methods of directly or indirectly teaching patients to replace their disturbance with some new skills, attitudes, thoughts, emotions, or behavior. This strategy falls back on a primary principle of operant learning theory. The best way to decrease undesirable behavior is not punishment but the building and reinforcement of a new, more adaptive response. In REBT, psychotherapists help the patient adopt alternative RBs that are based on Stoic and other philosophies. REBT also helps patients replace their disturbed negative emotions with non-disturbed negative emotions and replace their dysfunctional behavior with more adaptive ones. CT encourages the construction of adaptive automatic thoughts that are consistent with empirical reality and new adaptive schema that more accurately reflect reality. ACT does not attempt to change the content of beliefs or reduce the intensity or type of emotions. Instead, ACT teaches clients to learn to have a new flexible connection between thoughts or emotions and adaptive behaviors. DBT attempts to teach patients a philosophy of acceptance and teaches skills in emotion regulation through discomfort, diffusion, and changing the content of their thoughts.

Expression and experience of emotions in the session

Research has demonstrated that, regardless of theoretical orientation, encouraging patients to experience and express emotions in therapy is related to better psychotherapy outcomes (Peluso & Freund, 2019). All forms of CBT use techniques that increase the experience of emotions during therapy sessions. Encouraging emotions will increase the likelihood of linking patients' negative emotions to their IBs, negative thoughts, schema, and avoidance reactions. This information helps the psychotherapist understand the patient better and develop a more accurate case conceptualization. For REBT and CT, the depth, permanence, and effectiveness of evaluating thoughts and beliefs are enhanced when performed in the context of heightened emotional arousal. For ACT and DBT, the expression of difficult emotions provides direct exposure to the emotion. It directly is linked to the goal of reducing experiential avoidance, leading to greater psychological flexibility. Thus, all CBT models appear to focus on fostering experiencing emotions during psychotherapy.

Characteristic treatment techniques

All CBT models focus on changing patients' present thoughts, emotions, or behaviors. Most therapy models attempt to change clients' thoughts, emotions, and behaviors. In contrast, ACT attempts to get clients to change only their behaviors in the face of dysfunctional thoughts and distressing emotions. All such endeavors require clients to try new thoughts, emotions, or behaviors. And the therapists must convince clients to implement the change. Therapists use some form of education or persuasion strategy to convince the client to change. REBT does this by using Socratic dialogue and didactic teaching. REBT employs the frequent use of metaphors, parables, and humor as agents of change. Also, REBT practitioners use role-playing and psychoeducation. Other CBT models also refer to using Socratic questioning, metaphor, and role-plays to achieve such changes. CT uses Socratic questioning as the primary strategy to test negative thoughts empirically, although other strategies such as metaphors are used. ACT uses diffusion as the primary intervention, but practitioners liberally use metaphors and experiential exercises. DBT also uses Socratic questioning, didactic teaching, and experiential activities. There are more similarities than differences in how the various CBT models persuade their clients to engage in new responses. ACT seems the most different from the other major CBT models.

Changing the content and sequence of interventions

REBT, CT, and DBT focus on changing the content of beliefs as the beliefs are seen as precursors of the emotional and behavioral disturbance. These models focus on the cognitions that occur *a priori* – before the fact – of the disturbance. They attempt to change the content of the beliefs that occur before the patient experiences disturbed emotions or behaviors. ACT does not focus on changing the content of beliefs but on changing the connection between patients' thoughts, emotions and their behavior, and increasing clients' willingness to experience distressing thoughts/feelings and engage in valued behavior when these thoughts and emotions occur (diffusion). ACT interventions focus on the *post hoc* – after the fact – connections between the distressing thoughts, emotions and behavior. This focus is a significant difference within the CBT models.

Developing the therapeutic alliance

As noted above, the therapeutic alliance consists of seeking agreement on therapy goals, attaining agreement on therapy tasks, and developing a bond between the patient and psychotherapist. All CBT models appear to place equal emphasis on seeking agreement to the therapeutic goals. However, differences appear to exist in establishing agreement on the tasks of therapy. REBT, CT, and DBT teach patients about the proposed mechanism of change and seek consensus on therapy tasks. The purposes of the activities are explained and linked to the patient's goals and the rationale for the problem and the treatment. The role of attaining agreement on the task of therapy is harder to identify in ACT. Our reading of the ACT literature and observations of ACT videos failed to uncover specific discussion of or a rationale for why these tasks are relevant to relieving patients' problems. While watching ACT videos in class, my students expressed confusion and say they fail to see the therapist provide an understandable rationale for the intervention to the client. They also report personally failing to understand the rationale for the therapist's interventions. I agreed with the students. The ACT videos fail to provide clients with a convincing explanation for the therapeutic tasks or seek agreement to engage in the therapeutic tasks. It appears that seeking an agreement on therapy tasks and providing a convincing explanation of the therapeutic tasks are not stressed in ACT. Why would the originators of ACT avoid such common factors of psychotherapy achieved by so many other models? Hayes (2012) proposed that teaching people to follow rules leads to rigid, dysfunctional behaviors. Explaining the rationale for a therapeutic task could lead to the clients seeing the intervention as a rule, following it too rigidly, and thus developing disturbed behavior. Therefore, ACT fails to explain the rationale for the tasks because they fear that suggesting certain activities are preferred could lead to a rigid rule. Clients would then respond to external stimuli inflexibly, leading to disturbance.

DBT was developed to treat Borderline Personality Disorder (BPD) patients who are noted for their difficulty in sustaining the therapeutic alliance (Linehan, 2020). Linehan (2020) indicated that a cognitive approach to therapy that questioned negative automatic thoughts was upsetting to many borderline patients because they experienced this therapeutic strategy as the therapist doubting the truth of the abuse that they had experienced. Questioning the validity of negative experiences is referred to as invalidating the experience, and validating the experience represents recognizing that an adverse event or emotion has occurred. The invalidating experience that BPD patients often experience from abuse perpetrators or their defenders results in the clients being more likely to develop a negative reaction to attempts to question their inferences and thoughts about their abuse. Linehan (2020) reported that this was the exact aspect of CBT that interfered with BPD patients' therapeutic alliance. DBT believes the validation of the patients' adverse life experiences is crucial. Such validation is an ongoing component throughout treatment. Although there are no direct comparisons of which form of CBT develops the best therapeutic alliance, DBT might be the winner, and all therapists might want to validate patients' experience as prescribed by DBT. Perhaps the REBT strategy to avoid targeting automatic thoughts for change has an additional positive effect of validating patients' experiences and benefiting the therapeutic alliance.

A philosophy of acceptance

Acceptance has always been an essential, distinctive feature of REBT. Searching *PsycInfo* for "Acceptance" in the TITLE with the terms "psychotherapy or therapy, or treatment or intervention" appearing in the text resulted in 6,711 citations involving acceptance. Searching for those terms in the ABSTRACT resulted in 45,734 citations. Although Ellis was not the first author to use the word "acceptance," he has done much to promote the importance of acceptance in achieving mental health.

Ellis has referred to several types of acceptance. The first is acceptance of reality. The world is as it is, and we can better create a way to live in the world if we acknowledge how the world is. Such acceptance might lead to finding better ways to change the world to our liking or ways to live with it.

Second, Ellis advocated accepting others, which acknowledges that other people are as they are and not as we want them to be. The importance of acceptance of others has become a key component in couples therapy, where accepting one's partner is a significant part of therapy, as exemplified in the work of Christensen et al. (2020).

Third, Ellis advocated for acceptance of our subjective experience, which is our disturbing thoughts and emotions. Not accepting our subjective experience leads to meta-disturbance and many dysfunctional avoidance behaviors. Ellis also coined a term for the emotion that is generated by nonacceptance of our subjective experiences – discomfort anxiety. As noted above, many other forms of CBT have adapted acceptance of our human disturbance.

The fourth type of acceptance is unconditional self-acceptance or USA. REBT appears quite unique in this regard. Most psychotherapy approaches make efforts to increase clients' self-esteem. That is, they help people to recognize their positive traits and behaviors, encourage them to think more positively about themselves, and to feel better about themselves. REBT maintains that such approaches to increase self-esteem are flawed. People will always make a mistake. They always have some limitations. They will always have some faults, and finally some newcomers can eclipse their skills. Instead of convincing ourselves to have better self-esteem, REBT advocates that we learn to accept ourself with all our faults (Ellis, 2005). In REBT, people are valued human beings because they exist, not because of any trait, characteristics, or performance. Once people accomplish USA, they can still rate their performance and work hard to improve a particular behavior.

ACT (which has the term acceptance in its name) and DBT place a strong emphasis on acceptance. However, we found that these modern, third-wave therapies utilize the concept of accepting one's subjective experiences. They put little emphasis on or mention the other types of acceptance. Thus, acceptance is both a distinctive feature of REBT, a common component of other forms of CBT, and a unique characteristic of REBT, depending on which aspect of acceptance you are considering. Acceptance of others and developing a noncondemning stance towards our transgressors are also distinctive features of REBT and some anger management procedures. However, other CBT approaches rarely mention it. Self- acceptance appears to be a unique feature of REBT and is discussed below.

Rigidity is the core of psychological disturbance

REBT posits that rigidity is the core foundation of emotional disturbance, and flexibility is the hallmark of psychological adjustment. These ideas are no longer unique to REBT but represent a central theoretical point of ACT and third-wave theories. REBT and some forms of psychotherapy promote flexibility in thinking, choice of emotional experience, and behavior that is conducive to positive mental health. Although REBT and other CBTs advocate flexibility as an aspect of psychological health, they differ in a crucial way. REBT focuses more on the destructive aspect of cognitive in flexibility. It maintains that if people give up their rigidly held IBs, they will experience healthier emotions and have greater flexibility. ACT and other third-wave therapies focus more on behavioral flexibility (Follette & Hazlett-Stevens, 2016). They primarily teach clients to rehearse a broader range of behaviors in reaction to their disturbing thoughts and emotions.

What aspects of REBT are unique?

Despite the similarities that REBT shares with all psychotherapies and with other CBT models, in particular, REBT does have some distinctive features that are unique to it.

REBT as a philosophy of life[2]

REBT has the goal not only of decreasing emotional suffering but also of increasing positive functioning. Ellis's writings can be considered a manual for a philosophy of life; he (Ellis, 1994) dedicated an entire chapter in *Reason and Emotion in Psychotherapy* to using REBT to live a happier life. Bernard et al. (2010) have explained how Ellis's work presented a foundation for the emerging field of Positive Psychology. Stoic beliefs are at the core of REBT's attempt to promote positive mental health and well-being.

Over the years, other CBT theories have modeled REBT's stance on promoting the good life. For example, although DBT was created to treat patients with BPD, Linehan's (2020) most recent book stresses the promotion of positivity, as reflected in its title: *Building a Meaningful Life*. Hayes makes a similar statement concerning the goals of ACT, whose purpose focused on "establishing a more open, aware, and active approach to living, and...their positive effects occur because of changes in these processes" (Hayes et al., 2011, p. 141). The Cognitive Therapy model (A. Beck & Haigh, 2014; J Beck, 2021) provides little discussion of using its procedures and strategies to achieve positive well-being and focuses almost exclusively on ameliorating psychological disorders.

REBT's foundation in Stoic philosophy provides it with another advantage. Once a therapist challenges dysfunctional cognition, they face the task of helping the client identify a replacement for the patient's disturbed one.

REBT has the most precise theory concerning which adaptive beliefs promote positive mental health and reduce emotional disturbance. Each IB has a corresponding adaptive RB that is rooted in Stoic philosophy.

Imperatives versus thoughts concerning the occurrence of negative events

Perhaps the most distinctive feature of REBT, and the one most confusing to non-REBT psychotherapists, is the distinction between the elegant and the inelegant solutions. This distinction involves which cognitions psychotherapists target for change. David and Szentágotai (2006) noted that any taxonomy of cognitions within the CBT tradition needs to include the fundamental distinction between knowing and appraising. Abelson and Rosenberg (1958) originally proposed the terms "hot and cold" cognitions to distinguish between appraisals (hot cognitions) and knowledge (cold cognitions) of presumed facts. "Cold" cognitions refer to people's thoughts about the occurrences of relevant circumstances (i.e., information that explains adverse activating events). In contrast, "hot" cognitions refer to the appraisal of such events. That is whether the events are fantastic, good, adverse, or awful, as well as imperative thoughts about whether these events should or should not have occurred. Cold cognitions correspond to Beck's automatic thoughts or cognitive errors, while hot cognitions correspond to the IBs identified by Ellis (1962), such as shoulds, awfulizing statements, global evaluations of human worth, and evaluations of frustration tolerance. Other cognitive models identify appraisals and rules (should statements); however, they are considered intermediate beliefs and do not have the same saliency and importance as they do in REBT (J. Beck, 2021). Most forms of CBT identify and attempt to change automatic thoughts or cognitive errors first; it is unclear how long the therapy progresses before they might focus on intermediate cognitions. Also, the concept of schema is accorded a central role in many CBT models. However, the definition of schema is unclear. They are sometimes described as broad, conceptual representations of the real world (Young et al., 2003) and sometimes as imperative and evaluative constructs (Beck & Haigh, 2014). Again, sometimes schema are targeted after therapists spend many sessions targeting automatic thoughts and cognitive errors. Only REBT appears to target the demands and evaluations first.

For example, a cold cognition might be the thought: "No one has read my chapter." Or: "No one likes my chapter." The "hot" cognitions would be the appraisals such as: "That means that I am worthless," "I cannot stand that no one has read it," and "It is awful that people dislike my chapter." The imperative belief would be: "People must appreciate the work I do." Ellis considered challenging the cold cognitions as inelegant because the patient could feel better as long as the cold cognition was an error or a cognitive distortion. However, this strategy provides no way of coping with situations where the cold cognition is true. Ellis considered challenging the hot cognitions as elegant because it provides a coping strategy, whether the cold cognition is true or not. To arrive at the elegant solutions, REBT practitioners usually avoid challenging cold cognitions and ask patients to assume or imagine that their cold cognitions are true.

The elegant solution remains the cornerstone of REBT. Using it might contribute to building a stronger bond between psychotherapists and patients because we are acknowledging the seriousness of the problems that patients face. It communicates to the patient that the psychotherapist is willing to confront difficult issues, which is one of the characteristics of effective psychotherapists. REBT advocates the elegant over the inelegant solution because of REBT's theoretical position that patients' inferences (AKA automatic thoughts) are driven by our IBs. A rigid, demanding core schema will generate distorted perceptions, attributions, and inferences.

Some controversy exists even about how to display the distinction between cold and hot cognitions within the A-B-C model. Both cold and hot cognitions are thoughts and would fall under the B in the A-B- C model. Usually, when therapists ask patients what they think while confronting an A or experiencing a C, they report a stream of consciousness "cold cognition" because IBs are implicit and tacit cognitions. Once the psychotherapist uncovers a hot cognition, it would be placed in the Bs column with cold cognitions. Having two different types of cognitions in the B column leads to the therapist doing the inelegant solution. One way to resolve this problem is to identify the cold cognitions as activating events. They hypothetically could happen, and thereby could be events. However, they are thoughts. Although the A-B-C model has survived since Ellis created it in the1950s, it needs revision. Providing some way to differentiate between the two types of Bs, cold and hot ones, would be the best solution.

Unconditional self-acceptance versus self-esteem

Although acceptance has become a popular notion in psychotherapy, few forms of CBT or other psychotherapy models extend acceptance to the self. As mentioned above, REBT appears to exclusively promote the idea that humans work not to rate themselves but to accept themselves as they are with faults, warts and all. Most psychotherapies usually replace this nonjudgmental attitude towards the self with attempts to increase the patient's self-esteem. In my experience training psychotherapists, this aspect of REBT is the hardest to teach and the easiest for professionals to miss.

Unhealthy negative emotions (UNEs) versus healthy negative emotions (HNEs)

Perhaps the most unique aspect of REBT is its position on emotions. Most psychotherapies posit that people experience emotions along a continuum and that disturbed emotions are those with high intensity. Correspondingly, moderate-intensity emotions are adaptive, and the goal of therapy is to reduce the intensity of emotions. Ellis maintained that healthy and unhealthy negative emotions are qualitatively different. Humans can have intense yet healthy negative emotions. In REBT the goal of therapy is to replace the UNEs with HNEs. REBT would advocate that when people confront an adverse activating event and think rationally, they will still experience a negative emotion that is helpful and adaptive in focusing on the problem and activating the person to cope with it. Suggesting to the client that they reduce the intensity of the emotion can be experienced as invalidating. It also might not help them muster the appropriate resources to cope with a severe activating even. This aspect of the theory has received the least research attention. Although some research supports this component of the theory (Moagoase & Ştefan, 2013), it needs further corroboration.

REBT as an integrative model of psychotherapy

Research has continually shown that most practicing psychotherapists prefer to follow an eclectic or integrationist orientation because they find that clients often respond to different interventions (Poznanski & McLennan, 1995). Since its inception, REBT has maintained an eclectic or integrationist character, and REBT could be considered the first integrative psychotherapy. When Ellis (1955, 1958) introduced REBT, he identified many therapeutic activities included in the model. These included unconditional acceptance of the client, psychoeducation on the role of thinking, emoting, and behaving, cognitive restructuring, emotive imagery, teaching clients about healthy rational philosophy, imaginal and *in vivo* exposure, and the use of between-session homework that included bibliotherapy, rehearsal of new social skills, and imaginal rehearsal of new behaviors, thoughts, and emotions. REBT posits that thoughts, emotions, and behavior are interrelated. By targeting the thoughts, psychotherapists can change patients' disturbed emotions and behaviors. However, the theory says that psychotherapists can use any strategy or technique that they find useful to change these beliefs. Clinicians can directly change the patients' behaviors through direct behavioral exercises that will change both the symptoms and the underlying IBs. This feature remains a strong reason for continued allegiance to REBT.

Ellis's longtime colleague Arnold Lazarus (2008) offered the most detailed discussion of a notion that he called "technical eclecticism." Lazarus noted that as long as a therapist had a theory and a good case conceptualization of the patient, they could use any techniques to change the underlying beliefs, attitudes, or behavior patterns that caused the disturbance. REBT can have a strong appeal to integrationists and eclectic psychotherapists.

Summary

In this chapter, I have attempted to identify the characteristics that REBT shares with all other psychotherapies and other forms of CBT, and its unique aspects. REBT includes many characteristics from the common factors model of psychotherapy. It shares qualities with client-centered and psychodynamic therapies. REBT has much in common with other treatments in the CBT family, and many characteristics of REBT have spread to other CBT approaches. The focus on meta-disturbance is chief among these. REBT has several unique features. Chief among them is the focus on the elegant solution and challenging irrational appraisals and imperative demands rather than surface-level cognitive distortion. REBT's dual continuum model of emotions appears to be its most unique feature.

Notes

1 This chapter is based on a keynote address presented at the Fourth International Congress on Rational Emotive Behavior Therapy, September 13, 2019, Cluj-Napoca, Transylvania, Romania.
2 See also Chapter 9.

References

Abelson, R.P., & Rosenberg, M.J. (1958). Symbolic psycho-logic: A model of attitudinal cognition. *Behavioral Science, 3*, 1–13.

Barber, J. (2016). Personal communication.

Beal, D., & DiGiuseppe, R. (1998). Training supervisors in rational emotive behavior therapy. *Journal of Cognitive Psychotherapy, 12*, 127–138.

Beck, A.T., & Haigh, E. (2014). Advances in cognitive theory and therapy: The generic cognitive model. *Annual Review of Clinical Psychology, 10*, 1–24.

Beck, J. (2021). *Cognitive behavior therapy: Basics and beyond.* New York: Guilford Press.

Bernard, M.E., Froh, J.J., DiGiuseppe, R., Joyce, M.R., & Dryden, W. (2010). Albert Ellis: Unsung hero of positive psychology. *Journal of Positive Psychology, 5*(4), 302–310.

Castonguay, L.G., Schut, A.J., Aikins, D., Constantino, M.J, Laurenceau, J.P., Bologh, L., & Burns, D.D. (2004). Integrative cognitive therapy: A preliminary investigation. *Journal of Psychotherapy Integration, 14*, 4–20.

Christensen, A., Doss, B.D., & Jacobson, N.S. (2020). *Integrative behavioral couple therapy: A therapist's guide to creating acceptance and change, second edition.* New York: Norton.

Damasio, A. (2003). *Looking for Spinoza: Joy, sorrow, and the feeling brain.* New York: Harcourt.

David, D., & Szentágotai, A. (2006). Cognitions in cognitive-behavioral psychotherapies: Toward an integrative model. *Clinical Psychology Review, 26*(3), 284–298. https://doi.org/10.1016/j.cpr.2005.09.003

DiGiuseppe, R., Doyle, K.A., Dryden, W., & Backx, W. (2014). *A practitioner's guide to Rational Emotive Behavior Therapy, third edition.* New York: Oxford University Press.

DiGiuseppe, R., Leaf, R., & Linscott, J. (1993). The therapeutic relationship in rational-emotive therapy: Some preliminary data. *Journal of Rational-Emotive & Cognitive-Behavior Therapy, 11*(4), 223–233. https://doi.org/10.1007/BF01089777

Dryden, W. (2015). *Rational Emotive Behaviour Therapy: Distinctive features, second edition.* Hove, East Sussex: Routledge.

Ellis, A. (1955). New approaches to psychotherapy techniques. *Journal of Clinical Psychology, 11*, 207–260.

Ellis, A. (1958). Rational psychotherapy. *Journal of General Psychology, 59*, 35–49.

Ellis, A. (1959). Requisite conditions for basic personality change. *Journal of Consulting Psychology, 23*, 538–540.

Ellis, A. (1962). *Reason and emotion in psychotherapy.* New York: Stuart.

Ellis, A. (1964). Thoughts on theory versus outcome in psychotherapy. *Psychotherapy: Theory, Research & Practice, 1*(2), 83–87.

Ellis, A. (1980). Rational-emotive therapy and cognitive behavior therapy: Similarities and differences. *Cognitive Therapy and Research, 4*(4), 325–340. https://doi.org/10.1007/BF01178210

Ellis, A. (1994). *Reason and emotion in psychotherapy: A comprehensive method of treating human disturbances. Revised and updated.* New York: Birch Lane Press.

Ellis, A. (2002). *Overcoming resistance: Rational-emotive therapy with difficult patients, second edition.* New York: Springer-Nature.

Ellis, A. (2005). *The myth of self-esteem: How rational emotive behavior therapy can change your life forever.* New York: Prometheus Books.

Ellis, A., & Dryden, W. (1985). Dilemmas in giving warmth or love to clients: An interview with Albert Ellis. In W. Dryden (Ed.), *Therapists' dilemmas* (pp. 5–16). London: Sage Publications.

Follette, V.M., & Hazlett-Stevens, H. (2016). Mindfulness and acceptance therapies. In J.C. Norcross, G.R. VandenBos, & D.F. Freedheim (Eds.), *The handbook of clinical psychology. Volume II of V: Theory and research.* Washington, DC: American Psychological Association. The Associate Editor for this volume II is Bunmi O. Olatunji.

Frank, J.D., & Frank, J.B.(1962). *Persuasion and healing: A comprehensive study of psychotherapy.* Baltimore, MD: Johns Hopkins University Press.

Hayes, S.C. (2012). *Rule governed behavior: Cognitions, contingencies, and instructional control.* New York: Plenum.

Hayes, S.C., Villatte, M., Levin, M., & Hildebrandt, M. (2011). Open, aware, and active: Contextual approaches as an emerging trend in the behavioral and cognitive therapies. *Annual Review of Clinical Psychology, 7,* 141–68.

Hollon, S.D., & DiGiuseppe, R. (2011). Cognitive theories of psychotherapy. In J.C. Norcross, G.R. VandenBos, & D.K. Freedheim (Eds.), *History of psychotherapy: Continuity and change, second ed.* (pp. 203–241). Washington, DC: American Psychological Association. https://doi.org/10.1037/12353-007

Kahneman, D. (2011). *Thinking fast and thinking slow.* New York: Farrar, Straus, and Giroux.

Lazarus, A.A. (2008). Technical eclecticism and multimodal therapy. In J.L. Lebow (Ed.), *Twenty-first century psychotherapies: Contemporary approaches to theory and practice* (pp. 424–452). Hoboken, NJ: John Wiley & Sons, Inc.

Leahy, R. (2018). *Emotional schema therapy: Distinctive features.* New York and London: Routledge.

Linehan, M. (2020). *Building a meaningful life: A memoir.* New York: Random House.

Matweychuk, W., DiGiuseppe, R., & Gulyayeva, O. (2019). A comparison of REBT with other cognitive behavior therapies. In M.E. Bernard and W. Dryden (Eds.), *REBT: Advances in theory, research, and practice* (pp. 47–78). New York: Springer-Nature.

Moagoase, C., & Ştefan, S. (2013). Is there a difference between functional and dysfunctional negative emotions? The preliminary validation of the Functional and Dysfunctional Negative Emotions Scale (FADNES*). Journal of Cognitive and Behavioral Psychotherapies, 13,* 13–32.

Norcross, J.C., & Lambert, M.J. (2019). What works in the psychotherapy relation: Results, conclusions, and practices. In J.C. Norcross and M.J. Lambert (Eds.), *Psychotherapy relationships that work. Volume 1: Evidence-based therapist contributions, third edition* (pp. 631–644). New York: Oxford University Press.

Peluso, P., & Freund, R.R. (2019). *Emotional expression.* In J.C. Norcross and M.J. Lambert (Eds.), *Psychotherapy relationships that work. Volume 1: Evidence-based therapist contributions, third edition* (pp. 421–460). New York: Oxford University Press.

Poznanski, J.J., & McLennan, J. (1995). Conceptualizing and measuring counselors' theoretical orientation. *Journal of Counseling Psychology, 42,* 411–422.

Radosevich, D.M. (2009). Finding the MVP's: Most valuable psychologists [ProQuest Information & Learning]. In *Dissertation Abstracts International. Section B: The Sciences and Engineering* (Vol. 69, Issue 11-B, p. 7147). Ann Arbor, MI: ProQuest Dissertations and Theses.

Rogers, C. (1957). The necessary and sufficient conditions of therapeutic personality change. *Journal of Consulting Psychology, 21,* 95–103.

Rosenzweig, S. (1936). Some implicit common factors in diverse methods of psychotherapy. *American Journal of Orthopsychiatry, 6(3),* 412–415.

Shedler, J. (2010). The efficacy of psychodynamic psychotherapy. *American Psychologist, 65(2),* 98–109. https://doi.org/10.1037/a0018378

Wampold, B., & Imel, Z. (2015). *The great psychotherapy debate: The evidence for what makes psychotherapy work, second edition.* New York: Routledge.

Wells, A. (2009). *Meta-cognitive therapy for anxiety and depression*. New York: Guilford.

Woods, P.J., & Ellis, A. (1996). Supervision in rational emotive behavior therapy. *Journal of Rational-Emotive & Cognitive-Behavior Therapy*, 14(2), 135–152. https://doi.org/10.1007/BF02238187

Young, J.E., Klosko, J.S., & Weishaar, M.E. (2003). *Schema therapy: A practitioner's guide*. New York: Guilford Press.

Chapter 3

Capturing and making use of the moment[1]

REBT-informed single-session therapy

Windy Dryden

In this chapter, I will discuss single-session therapy (SST) which is a way of thinking about and delivering therapy services. In doing so, I will show how well the ideas that inform the practice of SST fit with those that inform the practice of REBT, outline what an REBT-informed single-session therapy looks like in practice (Dryden, 2019a) and present a transcript (with commentary) of a single session of REBT-informed SST.

An introduction to single-session therapy

Single-session therapy (SST) can be defined as an intentional endeavour where therapist and client agree to work together to see if the former can help the client deal with their problem in one session, knowing that more help is available if needed (Dryden, 2019a, 2019b, 2020). As this definition shows, during the course of a single session, or at its conclusion, it may become apparent that the client needs additional therapeutic help. If this is the case, further therapy is offered to the person, unless it is specifically indicated that such help is not available. There are, in fact, occasions when the REB therapist might only have one session with a person. First, the client may state at the outset that, for whatever reason, they just want to have one session of therapy. In which case, if the therapist chooses to proceed, then it will be on that basis. Second, when an REB therapist does a demonstration, that will be the only time they will meet with the person. Albert Ellis used to do such demonstrations at his Friday Night Workshops and during his training courses and did so throughout his career. Incidentally, even in his therapy sessions, Albert Ellis practised REBT without assuming that a client would return.

Reasons why SST is offered

There are a number of reasons why therapy agencies offer single-session therapy to clients as part of their service delivery. First, SST reflects how

DOI: 10.4324/9781003081593-4

many clients behave when making use of therapeutic services. Thus, data collected from public and non-profit therapy agencies from around the world show that the modal number of sessions people have is one (Brown & Jones, 2005; Hoyt & Talmon, 2014; Young, 2018). Data also show that between 70% and 80% of those who have a single session are satisfied with it given their current circumstances (Hoyt & Talmon, 2014; Talmon, 1990). Also, about 50% of these single-session clients do not require further help after the session (Young, 2018).

However, perhaps the most compelling reason why SST is offered is that it is based on providing help at the point of need rather than at the point of availability. Public and non-profit agencies tend to struggle with waiting lists and try to solve this problem by offering 'blocks' of therapy sessions which are relatively unsuccessful. By contrast, SST both meets the needs of clients who want a rapid response to a pressing concern and reduces waiting lists and waiting time.

The goals of SST

As I made clear earlier in the chapter, SST is purposive and the goals of the therapist can be divided into outcome goals and process goals.

Outcome goals

The single-session therapist recognizes that different clients want to get different things from the session and endeavours to find out what this is at the outset. Some clients may seek emotional relief and hope to gain a sense of hope from speaking with a therapist, while others may wish to seek specific help for pressing concerns with which they have become 'stuck'. Sometimes being helped to take a few steps forward may assist the client to deal with the problem, which may enable them to travel the rest of the journey without professional assistance. Aside from helping the client to deal effectively with a pressing emotional concern, the therapist may be called upon to help the client to deal with a dilemma or to make an important decision.

Process goals

Process goals are those that are designed to help the client achieve their outcome goals. They are to be achieved in the session, in contrast to outcome goals which are be achieved after the session. One major process goal involves the therapist helping the client to identify a workable solution to their nominated concern which they might rehearse in the session, if possible. Such a solution may involve the client changing their perspective or their behaviour. Another important process goal involves the therapist helping the client to identify internal and external resources that they may use in implementing their solution. The final process goal that I will mention concerns the therapist helping the client to develop an action plan which will aid them in the implementation of their solution.

The single-session mindset in action

Single-session therapy is not an approach to therapy. Rather, it is a way of delivering services and a mindset which therapists bring to the work. Thus, SST can be practised by therapists from a variety of therapeutic orientations, including, of course, REBT. However, what is important is the presence of the single-session mindset when SST is carried out. This mindset has the following features which all have practical implications:

1. Since it cannot be known with any degree of certainty that a client will return for a second session, the SST practitioner works on the assumption that this may be the only session that they may have with the client. As such, the therapist works with the client to help them fully to address their nominated concern in the session on the understanding that further help is available to the client, if needed.
2. The therapist creates a realistic expectation of what can be achieved in the session, detailing, if appropriate, what they can do and what they can't do.
3. The therapist encourages the client to specify what they would like to walk away with at the end of the session.
4. The therapist and the client agree on a focus for the session and the therapist helps the client to keep on track.
5. As noted above, the therapist adopts a resources-based focus, helping the client to identify and utilize inner strengths and helpful aspects of their environment while addressing their nominated concern.
6. Having understood the nominated concern, the therapist invites the client to use all relevant information to select the most feasible solution to this concern and to rehearse this solution in the session. The therapist then helps the client to develop an action plan to implement the solution.
7. The therapist encourages the client to summarize the session and to articulate what they are going to take away from it. Then the therapist reminds the client that they can access further help, if needed, and ends the session on a good note, if possible.

Good practice in SST and the REBT perspective

In this section, I will discuss what is considered to be good practice in SST and outline the REBT perspective on each point. As will be seen, in my view there is a high degree of consistency between the two therapeutic areas.

Agreeing the objective of the session

At the beginning of the session, the single-session therapist comes to an agreement with the client concerning the objective of their meeting and the therapist makes clear, if necessary, what they can do and what they can't do. This represents the value that REBT places on *explicitness* and it is certainly something that most REB therapists would do at the beginning of therapy.

Engaging the client quickly by getting down to work

The single-session therapist engages the client quickly through the work that they do from the outset. The SST practitioner does not do a lengthy assessment of the client, conduct a case history or carry out a case formulation because engaging in these activities is not necessary for the conduct of SST and, if engaged in, they would make the session inordinately long without providing additional benefit for either therapist or client. This is consistent with REBT's 'let's get down to business' problem-focused approach. After asking his clients a few standard biographical questions, Ellis would in the first five minutes of his first session with a client ask the client what problem they wanted to discuss with him and begin therapy with them at that point. In my view, this makes REBT and SST a perfect marriage on this point.

Adopting a prudently active stance

The single-session therapist is prudently active during the session while taking care to encourage the client to be active. The REB therapist is active in their use of Socratic questioning which invites the client to be actively involved in this dialogue. Even when the REB therapist is didactic at various junctures, they ensure the client's involvement by asking the client to summarize the points that are being put to them and to voice their doubts, reservations and objections to any of these points (see later).

Being solution-focused or problem/solution-focused

An SST practitioner is either solution-focused or problem/solution-focused. The latter elicits the client's nominated problem from their perspective before helping them to understand the factors involved in this problem (problem assessment) and thence to find a solution based on that understanding. In REBT, a distinction is made between a client's 'problem-as-experienced' and their 'problem-as-assessed', a viewpoint that is consistent with the practice of problem/solution-focused SST practitioners.

Focusing on goals

The SST practitioner is focused at the outset on helping the client to achieve an end-of-session goal and to this end the therapist helps the client stay focused as well. However, the single-session therapist may also want to discover what goal the client has in mind with respect to their nominated problem and to make a connection between the problem-related goal and the end-of-session goal. Typically, the latter is seen as leading to the former. Ellis (1989) was sceptical of the REB therapist asking their client for an end-of-session goal, arguing that this was a case of the therapist foisting on the client a goal that they do not have. However, Ellis's views were related to ongoing therapy and not to SST. Having said that, in his single-session REBT demonstrations, Ellis would not ask the client for an end-of-session goal.

In general, the REB therapist tends to use the *ABCDE* framework to help focus themself and their client on the latter's nominated problem and problem-related goal. In particular, the REB therapist would work towards helping the client set a goal with respect to the main adversity that features in their nominated problem. While the REB therapist would tend not to ask a client for an end-of-session goal, there is nothing in the theory that would rule out this practice and I certainly ask for such a goal as an REBT-informed single-session therapist (see session transcript below).

Being clear

The SST practitioner values clarity in all matters. In particular, they are clear about the nature of SST and what they can do and what they can't do. They also strive to ensure client understanding and agreement throughout the session. Finally, they are clear about the availability of further help and, if that is the case, how the client can access it, and they explain their interventions and the rationale behind them, whenever practicable.

The REB therapist strives to be clear with the client and is especially keen to ensure that the client understands key REBT concepts. Being clear is another example of *explicitness*, which is again consistent with REBT practice.

Selecting an agreed focus

Time is of the essence in SST and thus the therapist's main job is to help the client select a focus that is meaningful for them. Most often this will be a pressing concern that has been on the client's mind. While the therapist's main task is to help the client to deal with this concern, they will also look for ways to encourage the client to generalize their learning from the nominated problem to other areas of their life.

The REB therapist would begin REBT by focusing on the client's nominated problem and would later help the client to generalize what they learned from dealing with their specific problem to other issues. However, this would usually not be in the first session.

Adopting a strengths-based approach

The single-session practitioner does not have the time to help a client to learn skills that are not already in their repertoire and therefore the therapist needs to help the client identify and bring to the session what they consider to be relevant strengths. This principle places SST squarely with what are known as the strengths-based therapies (Murphy & Sparks, 2018).

Although there is no formally acknowledged approach that might be called 'strengths-based REBT', this strengths-based SST principle is not inconsistent with REBT.

Encouraging the use of environmental resources

In addition to focusing on a client's strengths (i.e. internal resources), the SST practitioner will also encourage the client to identify and utilize relevant helping resources that are available to them in their environment (i.e. external resources). These may include supportive people in their life and organizations that may provide relevant assistance and guidance.

While the REB therapist would largely help their client to identify and change internal factors, the flexible practice of REBT encompasses a dual focus on internal and external factors. It is both/and, not either/or. When the therapist cannot help a client to change internal factors, they will certainly help them, if possible, to change external factors.

Focusing on previous attempts to solve problems

The problem/solution-focused single-session therapist will ask their client to identify what attempts they have previously made to solve their problem. Having done so, they will help the client to build upon successful elements from these attempts and to cast aside those elements that were unsuccessful.

While the REB therapist tends not to ask the client for their prior problem-solving strategies, this would not be deemed inconsistent with REBT practice.

Asking questions

Most, but not all, SST practitioners make liberal use of questions during the session and this poses challenges for therapists who have been trained not to ask questions or to do so sparingly.[2] However, the liberal use of questions is quite consistent with how the REB therapist practises.

Dealing with doubts, reservations and objections (DROs)

It is important that the client in SST leaves the session in a positive, optimistic frame of mind. To enable this to happen, one of the things that the single-session therapist does is to encourage the client to identify and voice any doubts, reservations and objections (DROs) that they may have about any aspect of the session so that the therapist can respond to these DROs.

This practice is very consistent with what the REB therapist strives to do when they encourage the client to express any DROs they may have about REBT concepts or the REB therapeutic process.

Using opportunities to make an emotional impact

The single-session therapist strives to engage the client in a way that head and heart can work together, thus helping ensure that the work has an emotional impact on the client. When this happens, it increases the chances that the client will take away something meaningful from the session. The therapist, therefore, seeks to avoid two things: a) having a theoretical discussion with the client and b) a situation where the client is so overwhelmed with emotions that they can't think. In both these situations it is unlikely that the client will derive much benefit from the session.

The REB therapist is aware of the importance of engaging clients emotionally in the work as there is a danger that discussions between the two can be overly intellectual. I have written on the need for the REB therapist to guard against this and to make considered use of what I have called vivid therapeutic interventions (Dryden, 1986).

Refraining from overloading the client

The SST practitioner may want their client to take away as much as possible from the session, given the fact that they may only be meeting once. In doing so, the therapist may unwittingly overload the client with many 'helpful' strategies and tips. The danger here is that the client may take away little of substance from the session. To guard against this the therapist encourages the client to take one meaningful point from the single session that they can apply in their life. This is enshrined in the SST principle of 'less is more'.

The above position is consistent with REBT. Given that REBT is an educational approach to therapy, the REB therapist is mindful that their main goal is not to teach a client REBT concepts but to help them to learn these concepts. Given this, a client learning one meaningful REBT concept in the session is better than them taking away four concepts, for example, that are poorly understood.

Searching for a solution

Particularly when the client nominates a specific problem, the single-session therapist strives to help the client take away a solution to this problem. Such a solution will reflect the strengths of the client, any successful elements of previous attempts to deal with the problem and whatever concepts the therapist suggests to the client as potentially helpful.

The REB therapist strives to help the client to solve their problems by offering them an attitudinal solution. So, the solution-focused nature of REBT is consistent with the same focus in SST.

Rehearsing the solution in the session

Once the client has selected a solution, it is important for the SST practitioner to give them an opportunity to practise it in the session. This enables the client to get an experiential 'feel' of the solution in order to evaluate its potential helpfulness and to see if they think they can implement it in their life. Such rehearsal is entirely consistent with the practice of REBT.

Developing an action plan

Once the client has settled on a solution, the next step is for the single-session therapist to help them to develop an action plan to implement the solution going forward. Such a plan will be general in nature, although the therapist might help the client to select a specific way of 'kick-starting' the plan.

Being a cognitive-behavioural approach, REBT recommends the negotiation of specific homework assignments which can be reviewed at the following session. So, given the nature of SST, helping the client to develop an action plan is not inconsistent with REBT.

Ending the session well

If the client is to go away with a sense of optimism from the single session, it is important for the SST practitioner to help them end the session on a positive note. To ensure that this is done, the therapist invites the client to ask any final questions or to tell the therapist anything that they might wish they had mentioned when they look back later on the session. Finally, the therapist reiterates whether further help is available and how this help can be accessed.

While the above practices are not regularly done in REBT, they would not be inconsistent with REBT practice.

As can be seen from the above analysis, there is much that is consistent between good practice in SST and what regularly happens in REBT. Taking this idea forward in the next section, I will outline what an REBT-informed approach to SST looks like.

The practice of REBT-informed single-session therapy

The initial task of the REBT-informed single-session therapy practitioner is to agree with the client that they will meet for one session with the intention of helping the client achieve something meaningful that they can implement in their life in the knowledge that more help is available if needed. If the client wishes to proceed on that basis, then the therapist and client will need to decide if there is time and willingness on behalf of the client to prepare for the session. If so, then such preparation can be done over the phone or by the client completing a questionnaire which is shared with the therapist before the session.

At the beginning of the session, the therapist asks the client what they want to achieve by the end of the session and reminds the client that they are working together to help the client to achieve that goal, but that again more help is available if the client wants it. This will usually be determined by the client once they have implemented what they learned from the session and allowed time to pass to see what happens.

If the client wishes to discuss a specific emotional problem, the REBT-informed single-session therapist may help them to state their goal in line with the 'problem-as-experienced'. Then the therapist creates a focus that is centred on that problem and sets out to make an adversity-based assessment of this problem using the *situational AC* part of the *situational ABC* framework. Thus, the therapist asks for a specific example of the client's nominated problem, gets a description of the situation in which the problem occurred, identifies the client's main disturbed emotion (unhealthy negative emotion or UNE) at C and then identifies the adversity at A. In line with good REBT practice, the therapist then encourages the client to assume that this adversity is true. At this point the therapist helps the client to set an adversity-based goal in line with their 'problem-as-assessed'.

Then the therapist helps the client to assess the rigid/extreme attitudes that underpin their emotional problem and encourages them to see that they have a choice between the one rigid/extreme attitude with which they identify as most responsible for their problem and its flexible/non-extreme attitudinal alternative. In doing so, the therapist helps the client to see the relationship between this flexible/non-extreme attitude and their adversity-based goal.

Having underscored attitudinal choice, the therapist helps the client to examine both attitudes and to choose the one with which to proceed. This is normally the flexible/non-extreme attitude. This represents the 'solution' in SST terms. The therapist then encourages the client to practise this attitude-based solution in the session by using such methods as imagery, role-play or chair-work.

Next, the REBT-informed single-session therapist outlines the change process for the client. This involves the client rehearsing their main flexible/non-extreme attitude, acting in ways consistent with this attitude and doing both of these things regularly over time. These activities are specified in an action plan agreed between therapist and client.

At appropriate times during the session, the therapist helps the client to identify their strengths, resiliency factors, values and external resources which they can draw upon during the session and afterwards as they implement their selected solution in their life.

Towards the end of the session the therapist encourages the client to summarize what they have learned from the session and plan to take forward into their own life. They are encouraged to ask any last-minute questions or to tell the therapist anything that they need to say before finishing so that they can leave with a sense of completeness and hope for the future. The therapist may then invite the client to engage in a process whereby they reflect on and digest what they have learned from the session, act on this learning and agree to see what happens before they decide whether or not to seek further help. However, it may be the case that during the session it becomes clear that the client would benefit from more help, which is offered to them. Remember that SST does not preclude more help being available to the client.

Transcript of an REBT-informed single session

The client, Nick, volunteered for a single session knowing that this would be used as a demonstration for a course I run on single-session therapy. He has given written permission for the transcript to be used in this chapter and wanted me to use his real first name despite me offering to use a different name.

WINDY: Let me ask you, when you started to volunteer for this single session, what led you to do so?
[I begin this way because I want to know Nick's reasons for volunteering for the session.]
NICK: I've got an interest in REBT. I am doing a master's degree at the moment. I changed careers recently and, in that career, I don't know, I have some issues with authority and...I don't know, certain situations I find it very hard to communicate properly. I find myself, I don't know,

not having the confidence to speak up and I can recognize some of the behaviours are just not helping me out. So, when I saw the opportunity to have a session with you, I jumped at it.

WINDY: And, so, what would you hope to achieve by the end of the session?

[This is a typical SST 'goal at the end of the session' question.]

NICK: I'd love to feel more confident and keep my head up high when I do have conversations with certain people and, in meeting environments, feel more confident to speak up without feeling that I'm going to make a fool of myself.

[Note Nick's response. He has stated a goal that is not bounded by the end of the session. This is quite typical. Just because a therapist asks a clear question in SST, it does not mean that the client will answer it as asked.]

WINDY: And you hope to achieve that by the end of the session? Or do you hope to achieve that by putting into practice whatever we might talk about and that increased confidence might happen as a result of that?

[My response here is to 'layer' his goals and distinguish what he can realistically achieve in the single session and what this could lead to later.]

NICK: Yeah, I totally agree. I think it would definitely take some practice.

[Nick sees that there is a difference and notes that whatever he achieves by the end of the session will require practice.]

WINDY: OK, because I think it's important for me to stress what I can do and what I can't do, and, however much I could give you confidence at the end of the session or you get confidence, the confidence will come from implementing whatever we decide that is going to be helpful to you. So, is there an example of this that might be coming up in the future that would be a good illustration of the problem that you can think about?

[One of the tasks of the SST practitioner is to distinguish what they can do and what they cannot do. In doing so I reinforce Nick's point about implementation of 'whatever we decide is going to be helpful to you'. Note the words I use; I am emphasizing the joint nature of our work. Also, note that I have asked for a future example for us to focus on. This is typical in SST and also good practice in REBT. It is easier to plan for change when one is working on a future example than if one works on a past example and then shifts the focus from the past to the future.]

NICK: It's a little bit strange at the moment because I'm working from home. I could probably give you a past situation, if you want. Will that work?

WINDY: Yeah. The reason I ask for a future one is because it's easier to gear what we talk about to the future. We can certainly look back, but we've still got to apply what you can glean from that past example to the future. But if it makes sense to you to talk about, really, a good, clear example of that, that would be great.

NICK: Yeah. Well, I mean, there will be future ones. I do Skype meetings all the time and there's always one person in particular, when I find out I'm speaking to him, I do clam up and go a bit...

WINDY: And are you going to be speaking to him?

NICK: Probably in the next couple of weeks there will be a high-level meeting which I'll have to speak in, yeah.

WINDY: So, does it make sense to utilize him as an example?

[Nick responds initially by offering a past example. By going with him it soon becomes clear that there is a future example to be identified and I give my rationale for working with it.]

NICK: Yeah, definitely, if that's the way you want to go. Yeah.

[Nick responds by putting me in the driving seat concerning the choice of example. I think he may be a little bit 'REBT' star struck. Remember his phrase earlier: 'So, when I saw the opportunity to have a session with you, I jumped at it.' However, I want to put him back in the driving seat, which I do in my next response.]

WINDY: Well, it's what's most helpful to you.

NICK: Yeah. I mean, I'd like to feel that I could go into one of these higher-level meetings and feel a bit more comfortable, definitely.

[Nick alludes to the future so I go with that.]

WINDY: OK. So, let's imagine that you've got this Skype meeting with this chap and what's the context?

[I ask for the context to help us both understand the situation in which his problem occurs. This is the 'Situation' in the 'Situational ABC' framework.]

NICK: Situational – I'm obviously working from home, on a computer. I'm working on a major oil and gas project at the moment. The gentleman in particular, he's quite high up; he's at a manager's level. He's quite a confident kind of person, quite cocky, he's always butting in on the Skype calls and getting his opinion going. So, basically, I work as what you call a packer engineer instrumentation, so I have to give my feedback on anything to do with that. So, I'm called into the conversation quite a few times.

WINDY: How many people on the Skype call?

NICK: It can be ten, it can be thirty. It depends...

WINDY: OK. But it's not just you and him, in other words?

NICK: No. It's in a group setting. Very rarely just me and him.

WINDY: OK. So, in a couple of weeks, you'll come across this guy via Skype. Is that right?

NICK: That's correct, yeah.

WINDY: And, so, what would the problem you think you might experience be like?

NICK: Well, as soon as I see he's on a call and as soon as I hear him speaking, I start getting a bit anxious – butterflies and I start clamming up.

WINDY: What are you anxious about at that point?

[Having understood the context a little, I ask for Nick's problem and he responds with anxiety. I then ask for what he is anxious about. In REBT terms, I have found the situation, and his major emotion in the situation (i.e. 'C'); I have now asked about what he is anxious about, which is known as an 'adversity' in REBT.]

NICK: …I guess saying the wrong things. I'd like him to respect my opinion, but, I don't know, I'm not sure if I come across that way. I kind of clam up a little bit and underneath I realize that I do have the knowledge and I do have the experience, but, for some reason…

WINDY: So, if you weren't anxious about saying the wrong thing, what would be different?

NICK: I guess I'd come across confident and not be so worried about speaking during these meetings.

WINDY: OK. So, a number of dimensions there. One is that you mentioned about coming across confidently and the other thing is not saying something?

NICK: Not saying something stupid, really.

WINDY: Not saying something stupid, OK. So, which of those two is the biggest threat for you? Coming across non-confidently or saying something stupid?

NICK: I think probably saying something. I mean, I guess it's not just stupid. It's saying something that's incorrect.

WINDY: OK. So, saying something wrong.

NICK: Yeah, saying something wrong is probably the best.

WINDY: OK. So, what's the biggest fear for you with this chap?

NICK: Probably that. Yeah, probably saying something that's wrong and being shut down for saying it.

WINDY: OK. So, are you anxious about saying something wrong? Would you be anxious if you knew that you wouldn't be shot down?

NICK: …Yeah, I guess so.

WINDY: You'd still be anxious about saying something wrong even if you knew that he wouldn't shoot you down?

[In this sequence I am asking Nick questions to find out what his adversity is, which is the aspect of the situation that he is most anxious about. I employ a number of methods here: adding and subtracting elements, clarifying what I am hearing in his narrative.]

NICK: Yeah, I think so. I guess it's about I want him to respect me, I guess. I kind of get these feelings when I speak in these meetings that they're talking behind my back once I've spoken, anyway. It might sound strange, but I feel like they do.

WINDY: Saying what?

NICK: I don't know. Just putting me down or, 'He doesn't know anything.' I mean, I've come back; I had a ten-year break from this industry and

I've come back into it and the confidence has gone a little bit. They know more than me, sort of thing.

WINDY: OK. So, your basic anxiety is that you might say something incorrect?

[From what I am hearing this is Nick's adversity and the other elements he has just mentioned are his cognitive elaborations that stem from his anxiety. In other words, they are cognitive 'Cs' that stem from his rigid/ extreme attitudes towards his adversity of saying something wrong in front of his boss.]

NICK: I think so, yes.

[Nick's response is not as definite as I would prefer and I could have picked up on his tentativeness here. But I choose to go with it and ask him in my next response for what I call an 'adversity-based goal'. This concerns how he would like to handle saying something incorrect in the meeting attended by his boss.]

WINDY: OK. Now, what would you like to achieve about the prospect of saying something incorrect?

NICK: ... Well, obviously, I'd like to say something...

WINDY: Instead of being anxious about that, what would it be healthy for you to feel?

NICK: ... I guess knowing that even if I do say something incorrect, then it's not the end of the world, I guess.

[Nick's response is interesting here and is probably coloured by his interest in REBT. Thus, he comes up with what is known in REBT as a 'non-awfulizing attitude'.]

WINDY: And how would you feel if you believed that?

[Note my response. If he believed that, how would he feel? I know that he does not believe this, but I want to see if it is a viable solution. The only way I can do so is to have him imagine that he has conviction in that attitude to see what that would achieve.]

NICK: ... I'd probably feel a lot calmer, a lot more comfortable.

WINDY: Right, but you still wouldn't like it, would you?

NICK: No, definitely not. No. I want to come across as knowing what I'm supposed to know.

WINDY: And, in advance, it sounds like you would still be concerned about the prospect of not saying anything incorrect.

NICK: Definitely, yeah. We all want to come across...

WINDY: But you wouldn't be anxious?

NICK: I think if there isn't such a terrible side of things – thinking they're talking about me – no, I don't think I would be anxious. I think, if I could eliminate that, I would...

WINDY: But you'd still be concerned?

NICK: Yes. Yeah.

WINDY: OK.

[In this segment, I am working to help Nick see the difference between being concerned about saying something incorrect in front of his boss and being anxious about it. In doing this, I am attempting to link the realistic feeling of un-anxious concern, if you will, with his non-extreme attitude of not liking this, but it not being the end of the world.]

NICK: Naturally, yeah.

WINDY: So, you mentioned that you have an interest in REBT, didn't you?

NICK: Yeah. I've been studying it in my master's degree and I really like the sound of it.

WINDY: Whereabouts?

NICK: Staffordshire University. I'm doing a distance master's.

WINDY: OK. So, from the point of view of what you know about REBT, how would you assess what your belief is, because we know what your feeling is, which is anxiety, and we know what you're anxious about, which is saying something incorrect, but what do you think your belief, or what I call your attitude, is that leads you to be anxious about saying something incorrect?

NICK: I guess I'm putting extreme pressure and demands on myself to always be correct; I must always have the correct answer to everything.

WINDY: 'I must always have the correct answer.' Right, OK.

NICK: Yeah.

[Picking up on Nick's interest in REBT, I feel more confident about using an REBT conceptualization of his anxiety, here linking it to the rigid attitude that he expresses.]

WINDY: Now, have you tried to challenge that for yourself?

[Since Nick has expressed an interest in REBT, I want to determine if he has had any prior experience in challenging his rigid attitude so that I can build on skills that he has.]

NICK: Not particularly. I've tried it on a few other things, but not this particular one. I've saved this just for you.

WINDY: You did? OK. That's very kind of you. But, if I was to ask you to utilize your skills in other areas in this particular one, what would it sound like?

[Nick has had some experience of examining his rigid/extreme attitudes and so I ask him to transfer these skills to the present situation and attitude.]

NICK: Well, I need to create a more rational view that it's OK to be wrong. It's not the end of the world. I'm not, as I've worded it, a stupid person if I do get things wrong.

WINDY: Right. And how about the 'must'? How would you challenge the 'must'?

NICK: ... Well, I mean...just because I think I must, it doesn't mean it's right, it doesn't mean it's true.

WINDY: Right.

NICK: And obviously because I'm exhibiting not very helpful behaviours when I am in this situation, hopefully, by changing from a 'must' to a more rational, flexible viewpoint, then, hopefully, I'll...

WINDY: And what will that viewpoint be with respect to saying something incorrect?

NICK: ... It would just be I would like to be right but I don't have to be right.

WINDY: Right, OK. So, if you bring all that together and you rehearse the idea that 'I'd like to be right. I don't have to be. It's not the end of the world and I'm still...' what? What's your attitude about yourself going to be under those circumstances?

NICK: I guess, in a work context, I'm still a valuable employee that has lots to give, I guess.

WINDY: Yeah. And that you can still accept yourself whether you say things that are incorrect or not, that would be the additional thing, wouldn't it?

NICK: Yeah, definitely.

[From an REBT perspective, Nick's anxiety is based on a rigid attitude ('I have to be right') and two extreme attitudes that stem from this rigid attitude: 'It's the end of the world if this happens' (awfulizing attitude) and 'I'm a stupid person' (self-devaluation). His concern is based on a flexible attitude ('I'd like to be right, but I don't have to be right') and two non-extreme attitudes: 'It's not the end of the world if this happens' (non-awfulizing attitude) and 'I'm still a valuable employee and can accept myself if I say things that are incorrect or not' (unconditional self-acceptance attitude). Note that this latter attitude is half his contribution and half mine.

This is the solution that will help Nick to be concerned but not anxious about being incorrect in the presence of his critical boss. I am now going to ask him to rehearse this solution to see if it sits well with him. I decide to take him through a guided imagery exercise.]

WINDY: OK. Now, could you imagine rehearsing that?

NICK: ...Yeah. Yeah, I think I could.

WINDY: OK. So, let's take you through a rehearsal. You can do this with your eyes closed or eyes open. So, you're about to join a Skype call and you know that this chap's there and you start off being anxious because that's the usual way of the world. And then you say, 'Aha, I'm making myself anxious. I know what I'm anxious about. I'm anxious because I'm demanding that I mustn't say anything incorrect. No, I don't have to achieve that. I'm not a robot. There's always a possibility and, if I do, that will be unfortunate, and I can still accept myself. Even if he and others put me down, I can still accept myself.' Now, can you imagine rehearsing that?

[Note that, in this guided imagery, I present the realistic possibility that he will begin by being anxious, but that he can use his anxiety to identify

his rigid attitude, respond to it with a flexible attitude and remind himself of brief versions of his non-awfulizing and unconditional self-acceptance attitudes.]

NICK: Yeah, I think I could do that.

WINDY: OK. Now, what do you think, if you took the same attitude about the idea that you'd like him to respect you, how would you deal with your anxiety about him not respecting you, utilizing the same approach?

[Maybe I am asking him to do too much work here, but I wanted to show how he could generalize this solution to another adversity that he mentioned at the outset – his boss's negative attitude towards him.]

NICK: …Well, I guess I need to challenge, first of all, the demand that he must respect me. I need to…accept that, if he doesn't respect me… Well, I need to create an alternative belief, really, attitude.

WINDY: Which would be what?

NICK: That I'd like the respect of my colleague. If he doesn't, then it's not the end of the world and I'm still a worthy person, I guess.

WINDY: Yeah. You can still accept and respect yourself, even though he can't.

NICK: Yeah.

WINDY: Now, let's imagine you really believe that, right? And let's compare your strong belief in that more flexible philosophy, and we compare it to the rigid one that you currently hold about at least your anxiety. Which of those two philosophies leads to the idea that people are going to be talking behind your back and telling each other that you don't know what you're talking about? The idea that you must always say things correctly and you must get his respect or the idea that you don't always have to be correct and you don't always have to have respect? Which of those two belief systems is going to lead to that idea that people are talking about you negatively behind your back?

NICK: Definitely the first one, the one where I'm putting demands on myself.

WINDY: That's right. Now, the second one you might still think, 'Well, they might,' but then you also might think that they may not. So, in a sense, I think this shows, nicely, that when we have these rigid ideas, we're creating our anxiety – and the way you've been dealing with your anxiety, unfortunately and understandably, is the way of perpetuating it, because you've been dealing with it by staying silent.

NICK: Yeah.

WINDY: Incidentally, when you stay silent, you're really saying, 'I'd better stay silent because, if I do say something stupid, then that will be terrible. So I'd better stay silent.'

NICK: Yeah.

WINDY: But you not only create your anxiety; your behaviour, which is to stay silent, also creates the idea, this picture of the world, that other people are talking about you after the meeting and saying what a bloody dead loss you are.

[My goal in doing this piece of work is to help Nick see that his rigid/ extreme attitudes leads him to make highly distorted inferences that are skewed to the negative and that if his attitudes were flexible/non- extreme, these subsequent inferences would be more balanced. I would not have done this piece of work if he knew nothing about REBT and if we were not recording it. Knowing that he was going to get a recording and a transcript of the session later led me to take the risk. Overloading the client is a problem in SST and one that I am aware I have a tendency to do.]

NICK: Yeah.

WINDY: You see?

NICK: Yeah, totally.

WINDY: Now, do you have any doubts, reservations and objections to rehearsing these new ideas that we're talking about here?

NICK: No, not at all. I'd really like to become more confident in the work- place. So, no, I'll definitely give it a try.

WINDY: Right, and my guess is, the more you practise these ideas and rehearse them, you can rehearse them – God has given us the power of imagination, so you could always go through the idea and practise it on a daily basis and certainly before you go into the meeting. And, the more you do that and the more you speak up – because, by staying silent, that's going to be a problem – the more confident you'll be and the more prepared you'll be if you do say something incorrect, because you might.

NICK: Yeah, definitely.

WINDY: Do you know why you might?

NICK: ... Because there's no guarantee I'll always be right.

WINDY: Yes, unless you're a programmed robot.

NICK: Yeah. ... That makes a lot of sense. Yeah.

WINDY: OK. So, is there anything else about this that we need to talk about?

NICK: ... I don't think so. I think that was the gist of it. I think rehearsing it's a good thing. I think it will help me out a lot. Yeah.

[Developing an action plan with a client does not have to be elaborate. The main point is that Nick needs to rehearse his solution, which he does seem to grasp.]

WINDY: Now, could you generalize this to any other areas of your life? These ideas that we're talking about, are they generalizable to other areas of your life?

[My thinking at the time was that I wanted to help Nick to see if he could gen- eralize this solution to other areas of his life. We have dealt with the two adversities in his work problem – his anxiety about saying something wrong and his anxiety about the manager not respecting his opinion. Now I see if there is another life arena where he can apply his solution. Again, I raise the question about whether I am overloading him.]

NICK: I think so. I'm not the most confident of people. I can be confident, but I'd describe myself as not the most social, and I really want to be social with friends.

WINDY: So, give me an idea of how you can practise this new philosophy in a social arena?

NICK: Well, when you're in groups of people, there's always someone who's stronger, and I have this tendency just to let them speak. So, I think I could practise it a lot more in that environment and try and be a bit more confident, and accept that...

WINDY: And accept that what?

NICK: And just accept that I'm going to say something silly sometimes, but it's not the end of the world. I'm still me.

WINDY: Right.

NICK: I'm still worthy.

WINDY: 'And, if they take the mickey out of me,' what?
[Here, I provide an adversity for him to grapple with.]

NICK: Then it's up to them. It's not my problem. I'm happy with who I am.

WINDY: Yeah, although you'd prefer them not to take the mickey out of you.
[The 'it's not my problem' response leads me to reiterate the flexible attitude that he would prefer others not to 'take the mickey out of him'.]

NICK: Of course, yeah.

WINDY: Yeah, OK. So, the point is that this philosophy, although we're talking about it with your boss and in terms of authority. So, tell me a little bit – I am interested about this idea of authority. Have you had problems with authority going back in your life?
[I am testing a hunch here, but it turns out that I'm wrong. No harm done, I think?]

NICK: I don't think so. I've moved around a lot. When I was younger, I moved around a lot. I never had much stability in schools and stuff; I went to a lot of schools. So, I guess I never had a chance to actually build my self-confidence in social environments. So, I think maybe it stems from that. I'm not sure. But not particularly. In my previous experience in the oil industry, I never wanted to progress, I never took the opportunities, again because I guess I didn't feel comfortable with my own abilities.

WINDY: Right. So, you've basically reacted to being uncomfortable and not confident by playing safe.

NICK: In the work environment, yeah.

WINDY: Yeah.

NICK: ... Yeah. I mean, I've got a tendency to not stop. I like to continuously educate myself, try a new thing all the time. So, I think that might be my reaction to feeling I'm not worthy or I'm not at a high educational level.

WINDY: But it sounds like now you are; you're doing a master's. Is it an online master's that you're doing?

NICK: Yeah, it's a distance. We're meant to visit now and again, but, yeah, it's predominantly distance.

WINDY: And do you experience this issue on the course?

NICK: Not at all. I've absolutely immersed myself in it and love it. It's really something that's appealed to me for a long time.

WINDY: OK.

NICK: Again, there's not much communication between people.

[I am not very happy with this segment of the session. It does not really go anywhere and I run the risk of reducing the impact from the work Nick and I did earlier. So, I decide to bring the focus back and ask Nick to summarize the session.]

WINDY: OK. So, why don't you summarize the work that we've done today?

NICK: So, first of all we discussed and highlighted the problem. We found a specific example of a future instance of when I may feel anxious and we highlighted that the issues are probably stemming from the fact that I'm placing demands on myself to be correct in every situation in the workplace and maybe outside the workplace. So, to dispute that, we looked at the alternative, more flexible attitude and belief that we want to take and, by practising and rehearsing that using imagery prior to the events, hopefully, over time, that will help me develop more rational beliefs, which should, hopefully, change from anxious to concern, and accepting myself no matter what happens.

WINDY: Yeah. The more you do it, the more you get the benefit, and what will happen to your level of confidence?

[Although the focus of the session has been on addressing Nick's anxieties, I do not forget that Nick began the session by wanting to be more confident and bring this topic into focus at this point.]

NICK: I'm hoping my confidence in these environments will improve, yeah.

WINDY: Yeah. Again, the more you do it with a healthier, flexible philosophy, my hypothesis is the more confident you will become.

[Note that I link his confidence with rehearsal of his flexible attitude.]

NICK: That will be great.

WINDY: Yeah. So, is there anything that, if you went home and said, 'I wish I'd mentioned that today in the session' or 'I wish I'd asked that in the session,' anything that you want to ask now so that you can leave with a sense of closure and that this has been a good experience for you?

[The typical way to end a session in SST.]

NICK: ...It's really quite hard to think...I'm not sure, really. I love the idea of just accepting yourself no matter the situation. We've gone with the rehearsal side of things. Is there anything for self-depreciation that you'd recommend for rehearsal or techniques to use for that?

WINDY: Well, to recognize, I think, that there's a technique which you may know about – it's called the Big 'I', Little 'i' technique. The Big 'I', Little 'i' technique is that, when you say something incorrect, then that is a little 'i', and your big 'I' is composed of a whole multitude of these little 'i's and you may not like the fact that you've said something stupid, but it doesn't define you.

NICK: Yeah.

WINDY: So, you might want to go home and draw a big 'I' like that and then put little 'i's in there and carry that around with you and say, 'Yeah, that is the bit of me that I've just revealed, I've just said something stupid, but does it define the whole of me?'

NICK: Yeah.

WINDY: So, I might suggest that as an additional thing for you to take away.

[Asking the client if there is anything that they want to say or ask before we close is always a risk. I use the opportunity to give Nick an additional way of addressing what he calls self-depreciation. Again, I wonder if I am overloading him.]

NICK: Yeah. I'll give that a try.

WINDY: Alright. So, are we done?

NICK: I think so. I've found it very helpful.

WINDY: Good. OK. Thank you very much and all the best, and thank you for allowing us to record this and to actually show it on the course.

NICK: No problem at all. Nice to meet you, Windy.

WINDY: Take care. Bye-bye.

Notes

1 Keynote address read at the Fourth International Congress on REBT, Cluj, Romania, 13–15 September 2019.

2 For those therapists who think they can't do SST without asking questions, I recommend viewing the famous Rogers/Gloria video which is, in effect, an example of SST. See www.youtube.com/watch?v=ee1bU4XuUyg&t=686s (accessed 5 July 2020).

References

Brown, G.S., & Jones, E.R. (2005). Implementation of a feedback system in a managed care environment: What are patients teaching us? *Journal of Clinical Psychology, 61*, 187–198.

Dryden, W. (1986). Vivid methods in rational-emotive therapy. In A. Ellis & R. Grieger (Eds.), *Handbook of rational-emotive therapy*. Volume 2 (pp. 221–245). New York: Springer.

Dryden, W. (2019a). *Single-session 'one-at-a-time' (OAAT) therapy: A rational emotive behaviour therapy approach*. Abingdon, Oxon: Routledge.

Dryden, W. (2019b). *Single-session therapy: 100 key points and techniques*. Abingdon, Oxon: Routledge.

Dryden, W. (2020). *The single-session therapy primer: Principles and practice*. Monmouth: PCCS Books.

Ellis, A. (1989). Ineffective consumerism in the cognitive-behavioural therapies and in general psychotherapy. In W. Dryden & P. Trower (Eds.), *Cognitive psychotherapy: Stasis and change* (pp. 159–174). London: Cassell.

Hoyt, M.F., & Talmon, M.F. (2014). What the literature says: An annotated bibliography. In M.F. Hoyt & M. Talmon (Eds.), *Capturing the moment: Single session therapy and walk-in services* (pp. 487–516). Bethel, CT: Crown House Publishing.

Murphy, J.J., & Sparks, J.A. (2018). *Strengths-based therapy: Distinctive features.* Abingdon, Oxon: Routledge.

Talmon, M. (1990). *Single session therapy: Maximising the effect of the first (and often only) therapeutic encounter.* San Francisco, CA: Jossey-Bass.

Young, J. (2018). SST: The misunderstood gift that keeps on giving. In M.F. Hoyt, M. Bobele, A. Slive, J. Young, & M. Talmon (Eds.), *Single-session therapy by walk-in or appointment: Administrative, clinical, and supervisory aspects of one-at-a-time services* (pp. 40–58). New York: Routledge.

Part II

What REBT practitioners can learn from the wider world of psychotherapy

Chapter 4

Optimizing cognitive behavioral therapy to reduce the burden of distress disorders within an emotion regulation framework

Michal Clayton, Phillip E. Spaeth,
Megan E. Renna, David M. Fresco,
and Douglas S. Mennin

Distress disorders, including generalized anxiety disorder and major depressive disorder, remain a considerable public health concern. Moreover, otherwise efficacious treatments (e.g., medication and psychotherapy) tend to produce uneven or reduced treatment responses for these disorders, possibly due to core features of excessive emotionality and negative self-referentiality. To address these challenges, this chapter offers an affect-science based framework to guide the integration of common intervention processes into targeted mechanisms for the refractory features of distress. A functional emotion regulation perspective that emphasizes temporally consecutive motivational mechanisms, attentional and metacognitive mechanisms, and behavioral consequences is presented. We offer emotion regulation therapy (ERT) as an integration of traditional and contemporary CBTs (e.g., REBT), mindfulness, and emotion-focused interventions that reflect these mechanisms in the treatment of distress disorders. Clinical components of ERT are described, as are efficacy and mechanism findings from open and randomized controlled psychotherapy trials of ERT.

The term "distress disorders" refers to a subset of psychiatric conditions (e.g., generalized anxiety disorder [GAD], major depressive disorder [MDD], persistent depressive disorder [DYS], and post-traumatic stress disorder [PTSD]) characterized by the phenomenological experience of chronic and enduring distress over time. Aside from their shared observable characteristics, distress disorders pose a significant public health burden as they are among the most commonly occurring and impairing psychiatric disorders (Kessler, Berglund et al., 2005; Kessler, Chiu, Demler, & Walters, 2005). For example, lifetime (2.5% to 16.6%) and 12-month (1.5% to 6.7%) prevalence of these conditions is considerable. Distress disorders demonstrate a chronic and persistent course and are not likely to spontaneously remit without intervention (Tyrer & Baldwin, 2006).

DOI: 10.4324/9781003081593-6

They also complicate the presentation and treatment of medical conditions throughout the lifespan, contributing to both an increased risk of cardio-vascular disease (Cohen, Edmondson, & Kronish, 2015; Hare, Toukhsati, Johansson, & Jaarsma, 2014) and metabolic syndrome (Skilton, Moulin, Terra, & Bonnet, 2007). The burden of distress disorders is particularly prevalent among older adults (Wolitzky-Taylor, Castriotta, Lenze, Stanley, & Craske, 2010).

A recent study examining the world disease burden from all medical conditions in 2010 estimated that mood disorders were the second leading cause of years lived with disability (YLD) throughout the world (Murray & Lopez, 2013). Further, a 2010 study estimated that anxiety disorders (which included GAD and, at the time, PTSD) were named as the fifth leading cause of YLD (Murray & Lopez, 2013). Individuals diagnosed with distress disorders also are likely to engage in numerous health risk behaviors (Clancy, Prestwich, Caperon, & O'Connor, 2016). Individuals experiencing depression and anxiety are more likely to smoke tobacco, consume greater quantities of alcohol, be more sedentary, and consume an unhealthy diet (Strine et al., 2008). Findings have indicated that both veterans and non-veterans diagnosed with PTSD are more likely to smoke tobacco, consume alcohol, be sedentary, and be medication nonadherent compared to individuals without PTSD (Rheingold, Acierno, & Resnick, 2004; Zen, Whooley, Zhao, & Cohen, 2012).

Distress disorders can best be characterized by prolonged internal suffering, ranging from self-focused processing of negative emotions and stressors to intensely aversive and prolonged emotional states (Brosschot, Verkuil, & Thayer, 2018; Mennin & Fresco, 2015). This intense emotion-ality is often associated with attentional rigidity in processing both intero-ceptive and exteroceptive emotional stimuli (Clasen, Wells, Ellis, & Beevers, 2013; Etkin & Schatzberg, 2011; Mennin & Fresco, 2015; Mogg & Bradley, 2005) and negative self-referential processes (NSRPs) including worry, rumination (Mennin & Fresco, 2013), and self-criticism (e.g., Blatt, 1995), which is associated with habitually inflexible and dysfunctional behavioral responses (e.g., Ferster, 1973), deficits in reward sensitivity (e.g., Bogdan & Pizzagalli, 2006; Forbes, Shaw, & Dahl, 2007), and aversive stimulus gener-alization (e.g., Lissek, 2012).

These core features of distress disorders, including excessive emotion-ality (e.g., Olatunji, Cisler, & Tolin, 2010) and negative self-referentiality (e.g., Michalak, Hölz, & Teismann, 2011; Watkins et al., 2011) complicate treatment response, and overall otherwise efficacious treatments (e.g., medi-cation and psychotherapy) tend to underperform in treatment efficacy. Meta-analytic studies of GAD (Borkovec & Ruscio, 2001), MDD/DYS (Cuijpers, Smit, Bohlmeijer, Hollon, & Andersson, 2010) and PTSD (Steenkamp, Litz, Hoge, & Marmar, 2015) reveal this unevenness in treatment response to efficacious psychotherapies such as CBT. Given the challenges posed by distress disorders, a comprehensive and multicomponent intervention is likely required to achieve an optimal and durable treatment response.

This chapter offers a framework to guide the integration of common intervention processes into specified mechanisms that target the essential and refractory features of distress, including NSRPs. In the remainder of this chapter, we review: 1) how an emotional regulation perspective on distress disorders can bind these processes together in a functional model that targets specified mechanisms of change, and 2) how emotion regulation therapy (ERT) incorporates these intervention processes and demonstrates evidence in support of ERT as a treatment for distress disorders.

A functional emotion regulation perspective

The emotion regulation/dysregulation model

Drawing from advances in affect science, including emotion theory (e.g., Ekman & Davidson, 1994), emotion regulation (e.g., Gross, 2015), and affective neuroscience (e.g., Davidson, Jackson, & Kalin, 2000), distress-related conditions may best be understood as a failure in three temporally consecutive mechanisms (Mennin & Fresco, 2014): 1) motivational mechanisms (the initial response) that mobilize the pursuit of safety/reducing perceived threat, reward/minimizing loss, or both; 2) regulatory mechanisms (secondary responses), encompassing attentional (e.g., broadening, shifting, and sustaining attention to interoceptive and exteroceptive emotional stimuli) and more elaborative metacognitive strategies (e.g., decentering, cognitive reappraisal); and 3) behavioral consequences that include short-term maladaptive behavioral outcomes and long-term impacts on threat and reward learning. This model stresses motivational, regulatory, and behavioral mechanisms and emphasizes the temporal cascade of these mechanisms in explaining momentary distress within the distress conditions.

Motivational mechanisms

Emotion generation is functional and tied to our motivations (Keltner & Gross, 1999), which signal the importance of attending to, and possibly acting upon, a particular stimulus (Frijda, 1986). Although normative functioning represents a constant state of engaging and resolving conflict with reward and security motivations, individuals with distress disorders evidence a motivational imbalance that prioritizes safety at the expense of reward (Klenk, Strauman, & Higgins, 2011), thereby increasing levels of subjective intensity and corresponding distress.

Regulatory mechanisms

Emotions are part of a larger self-regulation system that involves coordination across numerous biological and behavioral systems, which allows us to flexibly respond to events in our lives in accordance with changing contexts and personal goals/values (Bonanno, Papa, Lalande, Westphal, & Coifman, 2004; Keltner & Gross, 1999; Wilson & Murrell, 2004) and helps us fine-tune our responses so that they are temporally congruent with the unfolding of this emotion generation/regulation process (e.g., Davidson et al., 2000). Building on Gross's (2015) temporal model of emotion regulation, the unfolding of emotion regulation can be differentiated by degree of elaboration, or the cognitive complexity required to engage a particular capacity. Less elaborative regulatory mechanisms include attention (e.g., ability to shift, broaden, or sustain attention from one stimulus to another as per contextual demands), while more cognitively elaborative regulatory mechanisms are representationally more complex and require greater effort and usage of working memory (Badre & D'Esposito, 2007). In the face of ineffective attention regulation, individuals with distress disorders may resort to more elaborative, perseverative, and often cognitively depleting strategies, such as NSRPs. Optimal emotion regulation may begin by first engaging less elaborative mechanisms, followed by engaging more elaborative mechanisms, as needed.

Behavioral consequences

Within distress disorders, strong emotions and NSRPs lead to a variety of maladaptive overt behaviors that reflect situation-focused antecedent strategies, including physical avoidance/withdrawal of feared or perceived unrewarding contexts (Michelson, Lee, Orsillo, & Roemer, 2011), as well as compulsive acts to engage in inappropriate or harmful reward or safety behavior (Schut, Castonguay, & Borkovec, 2001). Additionally, individuals with distress disorders often engage in response-focused maladaptive behaviors, including reassurance seeking, alcohol and drug use, smoking, dysfunctional eating behaviors and self-injury that, like NSRPs, can become negatively reinforced by their actual or perceived ability to ward off negative outcomes (e.g., Clancy et al., 2016).

The temporal cascade of these mechanisms

These mechanisms can be understood clinically as being functionally related along an emotional episode cascade. To more clearly illustrate this cascade of motivational mechanisms, regulatory (including attentional and metacognitive) mechanisms, and behavioral consequences, Table 4.1 provides examples of two prototypical individuals confronted with an emotionally engaging scenario: awaiting the possibility of an interview for an exciting new job in a new city. "Jane" typifies an individual who demonstrates optimal emotion regulation in the face of this scenario. "Joan," in contrast, suffers from distress disorders (e.g., comorbid MDD and GAD) and typifies an individual who exhibits suboptimal emotion regulation. As seen in Table 4.1, Jane and Joan exhibit different emotion generative and regulatory responses in confronting this exciting but stressful potential opportunity. Consequently, Jane is able to use this experience to inform how she will face future situations marked by risk and reward, while Joan disengages from future, possibly rewarding opportunities in favor of protecting herself from risk.

Emotion regulation therapy

Components of ERT

ERT directly reflects the target mechanisms introduced above by integrating various therapeutic processes into this affect science framework. These therapeutic processes draw from 1) cognitive behavioral treatments (e.g., psychoeducation, self-monitoring, cognitive perspective taking, problem solving); 2) acceptance-, dialectic-, and mindfulness-based behavioral treatments (e.g., mindfulness exercises to broaden awareness of sensations, bodily responses, and emotions in the present moment; exercises to increase willingness to accept emotions; commitment to action related to personal values; Hayes, Strosahl, & Wilson, 2012; Linehan, 1993; Roemer & Orsillo, 2009; Segal, Williams, & Teasdale, 2002); 3) experiential therapy (e.g., focus on empathic attunement, importance of agency, delineation of emotion function, engagement of experiential tasks; e.g., Elliott, Watson, Goldman, & Greenberg, 2004); and 4) brief psychodynamic therapies (e.g., motivational analysis, attachment history, focus on internal representations of relationships; e.g., Fosha, 2001; McCullough et al., 2003). ERT is delivered in a two-phase format with the collective goal of generating emotional clarity for action, rather than reactively and automatically being pulled to action (Renna, Quintero, Fresco, & Mennin, 2017). Figure 4.1 portrays the ERT model, including the components of Phase I and Phase II discussed in detail in the following subsections.

Phase I: Building regulation skills

Being counteractive

The first component of Phase I seeks to increase clients' awareness of moments when strong emotional reactions occur and the manner in which this cascade leads to action or inaction. This goal is accomplished through 1) psychoeducation of antecedents and consequences of NSRPs, including earlier motivational responses and later contextual/behavioral learning

Table 4.1 **Prototypical case examples of the temporal progression of normative and dysfunctional motivational mechanisms, regulatory mechanisms, and contextual learning consequences**

Situation: *Exciting but challenging new job opportunity*

Temporal progression	Jane (normative)	Joan (distress disordered)
First step: *Emotion generation (security and/or reward based motivation)*	Excited but cautious about this possible employment opportunity	Nervous about being rejected; desires employment opportunity but feels dejected about possibility
Second step: *Attention regulation*	Notices, but resists, urges to check for email from potential new employer while at her current job	Has difficulty not checking for new email in hope of a response from the prospective employer rather than focusing on work
Third step: *Metacognitive regulation*	After not hearing back, may utilize reappraisal to respond to negative thoughts	After not hearing back, engages in self-conscious processing (i.e. worry, rumination, self-criticism) around distress
Outcome: *Contextual learning consequences*	Uses experience to shape value system by attending to not only motivation to protect self but also taking further risks in service of rewarding career possibility	Disengages from contexts with possible reward due to risk management; loses opportunities to shape values from new experiences

consequences, reflected in thoughts and behaviors subsequently enacted; 2) self-monitoring and cue detection for online momentary analysis of emotional reactions and the functional use of NSRPs; and 3) gaining subsequent clarity and agency in taking actions that are most adaptive in a given context (i.e., "being counteractive").

Psychoeducation in ERT contrasts the challenges of distress with adaptive emotion processing and encourages clients to provide personally relevant examples that highlight how strong motivational impetuses lead to attempts to assert control with NSRPs, resulting in behavioral maladaptation and poor contextual learning. This perspective is notably different than the model employed in REBT, which views emotions as epiphenomena produced by rational (i.e., healthy emotions) or irrational (i.e., unhealthy

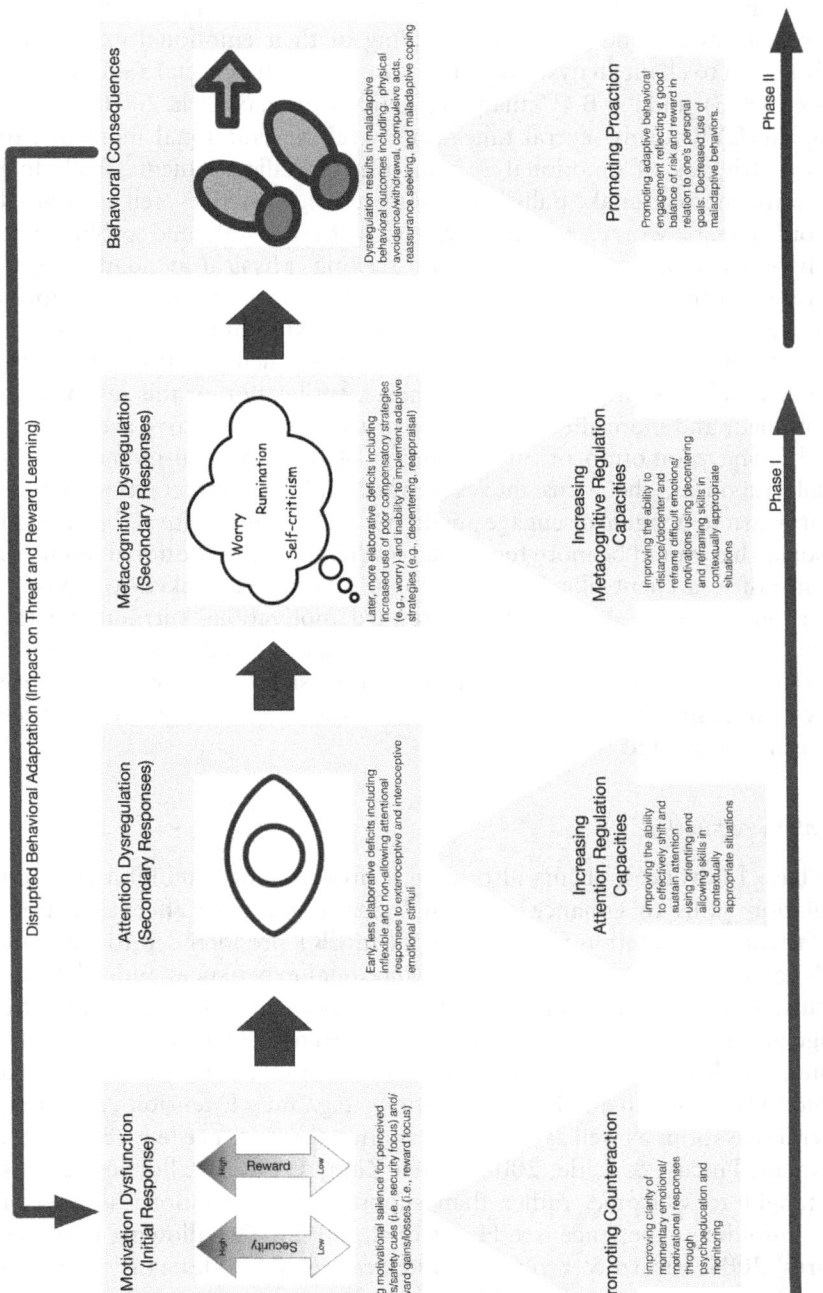

Figure 4.1 **Emotion regulation therapy model**
Source: © David M. Fresco and Douglas S. Mennin

emotions) beliefs (Dryden & Branch, 2008). In ERT, cue detection, referred to as "Catch Yourself Reacting" (CYR), helps clients gain awareness of the different elements and temporal unfolding of their emotional experience. CYR is akin to chain analysis (e.g., Linehan, 1993), functional analysis (e.g., Ferster, 1973), and "A-B-C" analysis (David, Schnur, & Birk, 2004). Clients complete CYR forms several times each week, in emotional moments, to identify triggers of emotional responses in specific moments, including emotions, motivational "pulls" (i.e., impetuses), "reactive" self-referential responses (e.g., worry, rumination, and self-criticism), and problematic behavioral responses (e.g., reassurance seeking, physical avoidance, compulsive repetitive behaviors, drinking, and self-injury). In session, therapists lead clients in a "Do-Over," which involves a vivid reimagining of an activating event from the past week to identify how their emotional response unfolded and how they can improve their identification of this response in the moment and more effectively intervene to produce effective action.

Following promotion of understanding of one's present-moment emotional responses, the focus moves towards taking counteraction, where clients learn to imagine or engage an alternative, "counteractive" behavioral response that would be more functional for handling an emotional moment. For instance, a client like Joan (see Table 4.1) may be asked to envision her strong security and diminished reward motivations surrounding the pursuit of a new job, and then to imagine what it would feel like with a different motivational configuration that emphasized her desire to advance her career despite the presence of risk, thus leading to a greater balance between security and reward.

Attention regulation

As Phase I advances, clients also learn a progression of mindful emotion regulation skills to enhance emotional clarity and take effective action. The attention regulation practices taught in ERT are intended to cultivate one's capacities for *orienting* to one's emotional experiences and *allowing*, or sustaining, attention on a particular experience. These two skills are designed to help identify and maintain awareness of emotions and the ensuing, underlying motivational pulls. In orienting, clients are taught to attend to their breath and bodily sensations (e.g., muscle tension), reflecting visceral sensations as well as their own emotional experience (e.g., Borkovec, Newman, Pincus, & Lytle, 2002; Kabat-Zinn, 1990). In allowing, clients are taught to welcome, rather than suppress, their emotions as part of their unfolding experience (see Hayes et al., 2012). The allowing practices (Marra, 2004; Ricard & Browner, 2006; Segal et al., 2002) assist clients in maintaining attention on the arising of conflicting emotions and encourage them to sit with this experience until they can hold and more clearly delineate the emotions and motivational pulls in the situation. This promotion of less elaborative interventions that do not necessarily involve verbal and higher-level cognitive knowledge structures represents a departure from traditional CBTs (e.g., REBT).

Metacognitive regulation

After gaining competency in attention regulation, metacognitive regulation skills are cultivated to utilize later in the temporal unfolding of an emotional moment. The first component of this skillset is decentering or *distancing* as it is described to clients. Decentering reflects a metacognitive ability to observe items that arise in the mind (e.g., thoughts, feelings, memories, etc.) with healthy psychological distance (Bernstein et al., 2015). This ability is strengthened as clients learn to gain both temporal distance (e.g., viewing inner experiences as temporary; Kabat-Zinn, 1994) and healthy distance (e.g. Hayes et al., 2012) from emotionally evocative stimuli. In both the formal skills practice and the in-the-moment implementation for distancing, the focus is on gaining perspective in time and space by granulating the constituent parts of the situation and placing them, externally, on objects in an imagined place in their mind.

The final metacognitive regulation skill in ERT is cognitive reappraisal or *reframing*, which refers to the ability to change one's evaluation of an event so as to alter its emotional significance (e.g., Gross, 2002). Clients are taught to re-evaluate a situation to appreciate and validate the presence of emotional pain and provide courage and compassion for such experiences (Gilbert, 2009; Salzberg, 1995), which is accomplished by developing and envisioning courageous and compassionate statements that the client imagines receiving from a trusted other person or an imagined version of themselves at a different time period in their life (Gilbert, 2009; Segal et al., 2002). Clients practice noticing their self-critical thoughts and learn to "soften" them as they arise, invoking these alternative, self-validating statements, which are typically written down on the back of an index or business card and carried with the client in a pocket or put on a smartphone, as a recurring reminder.

Phase II: Building behavioral repertoires

Being proactive

The goal of Phase II is to utilize mindful emotion regulation skills to facilitate taking proactions that reflect personally relevant goals and values (i.e., highest priorities and most cherished principles; Hayes, Villatte, Levin, & Hildebrandt, 2011; Wilson & Murrell, 2004). Clients are presented with different life domains (e.g., family, interpersonal relationships, community, self-care) and are asked to identify the relative importance of each domain and how congruent their lives are with the domain. Domains with a large discrepancy between their importance and how consistently the client is living by the value are optimal candidates for Phase II work (i.e., client indicates that the value is very important to them, but they are not living consistently with said value; Hayes et al., 2012). ERT promotes the importance of committing to taking proactive steps (Hayes et al., 2011), including a willingness to act in accordance with one's values despite the presence of strong security motivations, low reward motivations, feeling highly distressed from both strong security and reward motivations, or even high reward motivation without contextually appropriate security motivation.

ERT delineates three main exposure components to promote proaction, including: 1) imaginal action related to personally relevant goals; 2) experiential dialogue tasks to explore perceived internal conflicts related to the client's motivational configuration that may prevent proaction (Greenberg, 2002); and 3) planned between-session exercises wherein clients engage proactions outside of session. A number of modified, classic experiential techniques (i.e., imaginal exposure and experiential dialogue) are used to prepare clients for real-world exposure.

Imaginal proaction exposure

Congruent with traditional CBT interventions, such as cognitive rehearsal (Beck, 1979), in-session imaginal exposure tasks, focused on engaging proactions, are conducted to 1) provide the client with an experientially rich rehearsal of the steps that might be necessary to live by their values and 2) confront emotional challenges that are likely to come up as the client imagines engagement of proactions. In this imagery exposure task, therapists help clients imagine each step involved in engaging this action, while noting changes in motivational pulls and encouraging skills usage, to address difficulties in awareness and balancing of emotional responses.

Internal conflict exposure

The second component of in-session exposure work involves addressing perceived obstacles to taking proactions by using dialogue tasks. These tasks: 1) promote emotional tolerance when conflicts are experienced; 2) generate a new perspective (i.e., new meaning) on these obstacles; and 3) engage more adaptive emotions that are facilitative of proactive engagement. Obstacles are addressed through the lens of "conflict themes," primarily motivational conflict (e.g., security motivations are blocking or interrupting efforts that engage the reward system). These conflict themes are addressed within session using, in part, an experiential dialogue exercise congruent with gestalt exercises utilized in EFT (Elliott et al., 2004). Specifically, clients engage a dialogue between the part of themselves strongly motivated to obtain security and the part motivated towards engagement and meaningful reward, with the goal to arrive at a more unified motivational stance that is self-actualizing and conducive to proaction. Resolution comes when expressions from both sides of the dialogue demonstrate acknowledgement of the needs of the other and agree to engage commitment to the proaction.

Between-session proaction exposure

In between in-session exposure exercises, therapists encourage clients to engage planned proactions (i.e., specific actions taken outside of session related to salient values explored in session and committed to in the presence of therapists; Hayes et al., 2012) and to utilize skills, as needed, when they are planning to engage proactions. To further facilitate taking proactions between sessions, therapists can help clients to problem-solve external barriers (i.e., obstacles in the environment that are outside the client's control) that arise during exposure tasks. Similar to the CYR form, which is used to promote self-monitoring and counteraction in Phase I, the See Yourself Acting (SYA) form is utilized to facilitate taking proactions in Phase II. Clients complete the first part of the SYA form in session with the therapist to troubleshoot potential internal (i.e. emotional, motivational) and external obstacles to taking action; clients then complete the second part of the form after attempting to engage the action between sessions.

Evidence supporting ERT

Seven clinical trials of ERT have been conducted (three open trials and two RCTs have been published to date) focused on distress conditions (e.g., GAD, MDD) and distressing contexts (i.e., caregiving of those with cancer, COVID-19 impact). We offer a brief summary of the findings and will provide citations of published works for readers here.

Efficacy findings

ERT was originally developed and evaluated as a 20-session version in an initial open trial (OT) (N = 20; M age = 32, SD = 10.96; 75% women) and a randomized control trial (RCT) (N = 53; M age = 38, SD = 14.46; 81% women; ERT was compared to a minimal attentional control [MAC] condition; Mennin, Fresco, O'Toole, & Heimberg, 2018) of adults diagnosed with GAD with and without co-occurring MDD (Mennin, Fresco, Ritter, & Heimberg, 2015). Clients evidenced clinical improvement in the OT (within participant Hedge's g's = 0.5 to 4.0) and RCT clients receiving ERT demonstrated an advantage over MAC clients (between groups g's = 0.5 to 1.5). In both trials, ERT was well tolerated based on minimal dropout and gains were sustained for up to nine months post-treatment. We subsequently replicated and extended these efficacy findings (within subject g's = 1.5–4.0) using a 16-session version of ERT in an OT of an ethnically diverse sample of young adults (N = 31; M age = 22, SD = 2.48; 71% women; 55% non-white; Renna et al., 2018a). Beyond these indices of clinical response, an impressive percentage of clients in all aforementioned ERT trials achieved high endstate functioning (i.e., restoration of normative functioning) on a combination of GAD (Range = 55% to 85%) and MDD (Range = 56% to 80%) indicators that were maintained or increased into the post-treatment follow-up (Mennin et al., 2015; Mennin et al., 2018; Renna et al., 2018a; in preparation).

Most recently, ERT has been adapted for informal caregivers (ICs; e.g., family members, partners) of clients with cancer, who often report clinically significant symptoms of depression and/or anxiety that persist when left untreated. In an initial OT, 32 informal caregivers (87% women; mean age = 55, range = 61% partner, 19% children, and 16% parent of client with cancer) with significant distress and either elevated worry or rumination received an eight-session ERT adapted to the caregiver context (ERT-C). Caregivers receiving ERT-C evidenced considerable gains following treatment in worry, rumination, anxiety, and depression symptoms (within subject g's = .4–.9; Applebaum et al., 2018). A follow-up RCT in 81 ICs (75% women; mean age = 48; range = 75% were female caring for male clients) comparing the eight-session ERT caregiver protocol with a waitlist condition further found strong between-subject effects for these indices as well as a measure of caregiver burden (g's = .5–1.0). Further, clients whose informal caregivers attended ERT-C experienced a large increase in quality of life post-treatment compared to those whose informal caregivers were in the waitlist condition (g = 0.9; O'Toole et al., 2019a). In addition, we are currently conducting a mobile-based open trial treatment (video therapy and web app) of individuals directly affected by COVID-19 in the New York area and preliminary findings demonstrate high tolerability and strong indices of efficacy.

Target mechanism findings

These efficacy findings are encouraging but do not fully speak to the value of the treatment components in targeting the hypothesized mechanisms and whether these mechanisms account for positive outcomes. Thus, along with assessing clinical response, we have demonstrated evidence of changes in the putative mechanisms of our model (e.g., motivational awareness, attention and metacognitive regulation, behavioral engagement) with delivery of ERT using an array of biobehavioral assessment to demonstrate a relationship between mechanism change and clinical improvement.

For example, ERT produced attention regulation changes (i.e., increased orienting and sustaining attention ability) as indexed by behavioral task-related changes and neural correlates of decreased conflict monitoring during task presentation (Renna et al., 2018b, Seeley et al., under review). Also, ERT-linked improvements in resting state connectivity correlated with these attention regulation improvements (Scult et al., 2019). Regarding metacognitive regulation, ERT-linked changes in resting state functional connectivity patterns were associated with increased decentering and worry reduction (Fresco et al., 2017; Scult et al., 2019). Another study (Raab et al., under review) utilizing an explicit emotion regulation task (Ochsner et al., 2004) evidenced increased activation in neural areas associated with regulation, as well as corresponding increases in metacognitive ability and decreased MDD severity. Further, decentering and reappraisal abilities temporally preceded and drove symptom change in ERT (O'Toole et al., 2019a, 2019b). Findings also suggest ERT-related motivational change, as evidenced by decreasing negative implicit associations for approach versus avoidance over treatment, with associated improvements in life quality, functioning, emotional clarity, and decreased negative emotional experience (Quintero et al., in press). Finally, ERT-linked increases in parasympathetic activation following an emotion provocation task (a biological index of regulatory recovery from a stressor) were linked to decreased diagnostic severity, worry, depression, impairment, and life quality (Lee et al., in preparation).

Future directions/conclusion

Despite impressive efficacy, CBT's effects are not uniformly beneficial across distress disorders and these otherwise efficacious treatments fail to adequately treat a large subgroup of clients. In this chapter, we offered a conceptual model to guide the targeted development of treatments for distress disorders. For instance, ERT and traditional CBT share important elements, including cue detection, skills training, and exposure components. In comparison with REBT, for example, both orientations include a functional analysis (e.g., A-B-C analysis; David et al., 2004) that relates cognitions, emotions, and behaviors over time. However, there are also notable distinctions. In particular, a primary feature of traditional CBT, including REBT, is the identification and modification of distorted beliefs. This intervention principle emphasizes cognitively elaborative, verbally mediated, components (e.g., cognitive restructuring) to a greater extent than intervention principles that target less elaborative, attentional, components.

ERT also shares important elements with mindfulness-based interventions (MBIs; e.g., Craigie, Rees, Marsh, & Nathan, 2008; Evans et al., 2008; Hoge et al., 2015), which emphasize the targeting of less elaborative attentional features (e.g., sustained and flexible attention) via guided meditation practices. Although results from these MBI trials are promising, the effects on anxiety outcomes were modest and mood outcomes have largely been poor or minimal given that these trials excluded patients with comorbid mood disorders. Further, these studies have not examined clinical significance or changes in additional comorbid conditions.

Taken together, one possible interpretation of the relatively weaker comparative efficacy of traditional CBT or MBIs relative to ERT is that optimal treatment for distress disorders is achieved by interventions that simultaneously target less cognitively elaborative facets (i.e., attention) *and* more cognitively elaborative facets (i.e., metacognition) as opposed to focusing treatment largely on one or the other. For instance, the inclusion of attention regulation skills in REBT may facilitate monitoring and reflection on cognitions (e.g., irrational beliefs) that might be difficult for some clients to tolerate. Correspondingly, the above therapeutic processes can be understood as indicative of overarching change principles that directly target treatment mechanisms unfolding in a temporal emotional cascade: 1) motivational mechanisms; 2) regulatory mechanisms, which vary in their degree of elaboration (i.e., less elaborative attentional regulation to more elaborative metacognitive regulation); and 3) behavioral engagement mechanisms.

Future work will seek to identify the specific ways in which ERT skills contribute to ERT's efficacy by examining whether briefer, tailored interventions can more precisely target the purported mechanisms of action. For instance, an as yet unanswered question pertains to what is the optimal relative dose of attentional and cognitive interventions needed to provide the most synergistic treatment response? One promising way to potentially address issues of dosing for a particular intervention or even for a particular individual within an intervention is to utilize sequential, multiple assignment, randomized trial (SMART) methodologies (Collins, Nahum-Shani, & Almirall, 2014). Another important focus for ERT will be to delineate the longer-term impact of ERT on the individual's symptoms and wellbeing. ERT could reach a wider group of individuals through increased efforts at treatment personalization, including addressing specific contextual challenges of diverse groups in terms of race, culture, and socioeconomic status. Despite the need for these future steps, ERT demonstrates a novel approach for treating distress disorders in an effort to promote long-term ameliorative changes for individuals suffering from these conditions.

References

Applebaum, A.J., Panjwani, A.A., Buda, K., O'Toole, M.S., Hoyt, M.A., Garcia, A., Fresco, D.M., & Mennin, D.S. (2018). Emotion regulation therapy for cancer caregivers—an open trial of a mechanism-targeted approach to addressing caregiver distress. *Translational Behavioral Medicine*. doi:10.1093/tbm/iby104

Badre, D., & D'Esposito, M. (2007). Functional magnetic resonance imaging evidence for a hierarchical organization of the prefrontal cortex. *Journal of Cognitive Neuroscience, 19*(12), 2082–2099.

Beck, A.T. (1979). *Cognitive therapy of depression*. New York: Guilford Press.

Bernstein, A., Hadash, Y., Lichtash, Y., Tanay, G., Shepherd, K., & Fresco, D.M. (2015). Decentering and related constructs: A critical review and metacognitive processes model. *Perspectives on Psychological Science, 10*(5), 599–617.

Blatt, S.J. (1995). The destructiveness of perfectionism: Implications for the treatment of depression. *American Psychologist, 50*(12), 1003.

Bogdan, R., & Pizzagalli, D.A. (2006). Acute stress reduces reward responsiveness: Implications for depression. *Biological Psychiatry, 60*(10), 1147–1154.

Bonanno, G.A., Papa, A., Lalande, K., Westphal, M., & Coifman, K. (2004). The importance of being flexible: The ability to both enhance and suppress emotional expression predicts long-term adjustment. *Psychological Science, 15*(7), 482–487. doi:10.1111/j.0956-7976.2004.00705.x

Borkovec, T.D., Newman, M.G., Pincus, A.L., & Lytle, R. (2002). A component analysis of cognitive-behavioral therapy for generalized anxiety disorder and the role of interpersonal problems. *Journal of Consulting and Clinical Psychology, 70*(2), 288.

Borkovec, T.D., & Ruscio, A.M. (2001). Psychotherapy for generalized anxiety disorder. *Journal of Clinical Psychiatry, 62*, 37–42.

Brosschot, J.F., Verkuil, B., & Thayer, J.F. (2018). Generalized unsafety theory of stress: Unsafe environments and conditions, and the default stress response. *International Journal of Environmental Research and Public Health, 15*(3), 464.

Clancy, F., Prestwich, A., Caperon, L., & O'Connor, D.B. (2016). Perseverative cognition and health behaviors: A systematic review and meta-analysis. *Frontiers in Human Neuroscience, 10*(534). doi:10.3389/fnhum.2016.00534

Clasen, P.C., Wells, T.T., Ellis, A.J., & Beevers, C.G. (2013). Attentional biases and the persistence of sad mood in major depressive disorder. *Journal of Abnormal Psychology, 122*(1), 74.

Cohen, B.E., Edmondson, D., & Kronish, I.M. (2015). State of the art review: Depression, stress, anxiety, and cardiovascular disease. *American Journal of Hypertension, 28*(11), 1295–1302. doi:10.1093/ajh/hpv047

Collins, L.M., Nahum-Shani, I., & Almirall, D. (2014). Optimization of behavioral dynamic treatment regimens based on the sequential, multiple assignment, randomized trial (SMART). *Clinical Trials, 11*(4), 426–434. doi:10.1177/1740774514536795

Craigie, M.A., Rees, C.S., Marsh, A., & Nathan, P. (2008). Mindfulness-based cognitive therapy for generalized anxiety disorder: A preliminary evaluation. *Behavioural & Cognitive Psychotherapy, 36*(5), 553–568.

Cuijpers, P., Smit, F., Bohlmeijer, E., Hollon, S.D., & Andersson, G. (2010). Efficacy of cognitive-behavioural therapy and other psychological treatments for adult depression: Meta-analytic study of publication bias. *British Journal of Psychiatry, 196*(3), 173–178.

David, D., Schnur, J., & Birk, J. (2004). Functional and dysfunctional feelings in Ellis' cognitive theory of emotion: An empirical analysis. *Cognition and Emotion, 18*(6), 869–880.

Davidson, R.J., Jackson, D.C., & Kalin, N.H. (2000). Emotion, plasticity, context, and regulation: Perspectives from affective neuroscience. *Psychological Bulletin, 126*(6), 890.

Dryden, W., & Branch, R. (2008). *The fundamentals of rational emotive behaviour therapy: A training handbook. Second edition.* Hoboken, NJ: Wiley.

Ekman, P.E., & Davidson, R.J. (1994). *The nature of emotion: Fundamental questions.* Oxford: Oxford University Press.

Elliott, R., Watson, J.C., Goldman, R.N., & Greenberg, L.S. (2004). *Learning emotion-focused therapy: The process-experiential approach to change.* Washington, DC: American Psychological Association.

Etkin, A., & Schatzberg, A.F. (2011). Common abnormalities and disorder-specific compensation during implicit regulation of emotional processing in generalized anxiety and major depressive disorders. *American Journal of Psychiatry, 168*(9), 968–978.

Evans, S., Ferrando, S., Findler, M., Stowell, C., Smart, C., & Haglin, D. (2008). Mindfulness-based cognitive therapy for generalized anxiety disorder. *Journal of Anxiety Disorders, 22*(4), 716–721.

Ferster, C.B. (1973). A functional analysis of depression. *American Psychologist, 28*(10), 857–870.

Forbes, E.E., Shaw, D.S., & Dahl, R.E. (2007). Alterations in reward-related decision making in boys with recent and future depression. *Biological Psychiatry, 61*(5), 633–639. doi:10.1016/j.biopsych.2006.05.026

Fosha, D. (2001). The dyadic regulation of affect. *Journal of Clinical Psychology, 57*(2), 227–242.

Fresco, D.M., Roy, A.K., Adelsberg, S., Seeley, S., García-Lesy, E., Liston, C., & Mennin, D.S. (2017). Distinct functional connectivities predict clinical response with emotion regulation therapy. *Frontiers in Human Neuroscience, 11,* 86.

Frijda, N.H. (1986). *The emotions.* Cambridge: Cambridge University Press.

Gilbert, P. (2009). *The compassionate mind: A new approach to the challenges of life.* London: Constable & Robinson.

Greenberg, L.S. (2002). Integrating an emotion-focused approach to treatment into psychotherapy integration. *Journal of Psychotherapy Integration, 12*(2), 154–189.

Gross, J.J. (2002). Emotion regulation: Affective, cognitive, and social consequences. *Psychophysiology, 39*(3), 281–291.

Gross, J.J. (2015). Emotion regulation: Current status and future prospects. *Psychological Inquiry, 26*(1), 1–26.

Hare, D.L., Toukhsati, S.R., Johansson, P., & Jaarsma, T. (2014). Depression and cardiovascular disease: A clinical review. *European Heart Journal, 35*(21), 1365–1372. doi:10.1093/eurheartj/eht462

Hayes, S., Strosahl, K., & Wilson, K. (2012). *Acceptance and Commitment Therapy. Second Edition: The process and practice of mindful change*. New York: Guilford Press.

Hayes, S.C., Villatte, M., Levin, M., & Hildebrandt, M. (2011). Open, aware, and active: Contextual approaches as an emerging trend in the behavioral and cognitive therapies. *Annual Review of Clinical Psychology, 7*, 141–168. doi:10.1146/annurev-clinpsy-032210-104449

Hoge, E.A., Bui, E., Goetter, E., Robinaugh, D.J., Ojserkis, R.A., Fresco, D.M., & Simon, N.M. (2015). Change in decentering mediates improvement in anxiety in mindfulness-based stress reduction for generalized anxiety disorder. *Cognitive Therapy & Research, 39*(2), 228–235.

Kabat-Zinn, J. (1990). *Full catastrophe living: Using wisdom of your body and mind to face stress, pain, and illness*. New York: Dell Publishing.

Kabat-Zinn, J. (1994). *Where you go, there you are: Mindfulness meditation in everyday life*. Westport, CT: Hyperion.

Keltner, D., & Gross, J.J. (1999). Functional accounts of emotions. *Cognition & Emotion, 13*(5), 467–480.

Kessler, R.C., Berglund, P., Demler, O., Jin, R., Merikangas, K.R., & Walters, E.E. (2005). Lifetime prevalence and age-of-onset distributions of DSM-IV disorders in the National Comorbidity Survey Replication. *Archives of General Psychiatry, 62*, 593–602.

Kessler, R.C., Chiu, W.T., Demler, O., & Walters, E.E. (2005). Prevalence, severity, and comorbidity of 12-month DSM-IV disorders in the National Comorbidity Survey Replication. *Archives of General Psychiatry, 62*, 617–628.

Klenk, M.M., Strauman, T.J., & Higgins, E.T. (2011). Regulatory focus and anxiety: A self-regulatory model of GAD-depression comorbidity. *Personality and Individual Differences, 50*(7), 935–943. doi:10.1016/j.paid.2010.12.003

Lee et al. (in preparation).

Linehan, M.M. (1993). *Skills training manual for treating borderline personality disorder*. New York: Guilford Press.

Lissek, S. (2012). Toward an account of clinical anxiety predicated on basic, neurally mapped mechanisms of Pavlovian fear-learning: The case for condition overgeneralization. *Depression and Anxiety, 29*(4), 257–263.

Marra, T. (2004). *Depressed and anxious: The dialectical behavior therapy workbook for overcoming depression and anxiety*. Oakland, CA: New Harbinger Publications.

McCullough, L., Kuhn, N., Andrews, S., Kaplan, A., Wolf, J., & Hurley, C.L. (2003). *Treating affect phobia: A manual for short-term dynamic psychotherapy*. New York: Guilford Press.

Mennin, D.S., & Fresco, D.M. (2013). What, me worry and ruminate about DSM-5 and RDoC? The importance of targeting negative self-referential processing. *Clinical Psychology: Science and Practice, 20*(3), 258–267.

Mennin, D.S., & Fresco, D.M. (2014). Emotion regulation therapy. *Handbook of Emotion Regulation, 2*, 469–490.

Mennin, D.S., & Fresco, D.M. (2015). Advancing emotion regulation perspectives on psychopathology: The challenge of distress disorders. *Psychological Inquiry, 26*(1), 80–92.

Mennin, D.S., Fresco, D.M., O'Toole, M.S., & Heimberg, R.G. (2018). A randomized controlled trial of emotion regulation therapy for generalized anxiety disorder with and without co-occurring depression. *Journal of Consulting and Clinical Psychology, 86*(3), 268.

Mennin, D.S., Fresco, D.M., Ritter, M., & Heimberg, R.G. (2015). An open trial of emotion regulation therapy for generalized anxiety disorder and cooccurring depression. *Depression and Anxiety, 32*(8), 614–623.

Michalak, J., Hölz, A., & Teismann, T. (2011). Rumination as a predictor of relapse in mindfulness-based cognitive therapy for depression. *Psychology and Psychotherapy: Theory, Research and Practice, 84*(2), 230–236.

Michelson, S.E., Lee, J.K., Orsillo, S.M., & Roemer, L. (2011). The role of values-consistent behavior in generalized anxiety disorder. *Depression and Anxiety, 28*(5), 358–366.

Mogg, K., & Bradley, B.P. (2005). Attentional bias in generalized anxiety disorder versus depressive disorder. *Cognitive Therapy and Research, 29*(1), 29–45.

Murray, C.J., & Lopez, A.D. (2013). Measuring the global burden of disease. *New England Journal of Medicine, 369*(5), 448–457. doi:10.1056/NEJMra1201534

Ochsner, K., Ray, R., Cooper, J., Robertson, E., Chopra, S., Gabrieli, J., & Gross, J. (2004). For better or for worse: Neural systems supporting the cognitive down- and up-regulation of negative emotion. *NeuroImage, 23*, 483–499. doi:10.1016/j.neuroimage.2004.06.030

Olatunji, B.O., Cisler, J.M., & Tolin, D.F. (2010). A meta-analysis of the influence of comorbidity on treatment outcome in the anxiety disorders. *Clinical Psychology Review, 30*(6), 642–654.

O'Toole, M.S., Mennin, D.S., Applebaum, A., Weber, B., Rose, H., Fresco, D.M., & Zachariae, R. (2019a). A randomized controlled trial of emotion regulation therapy for psychologically distressed caregivers of cancer patients. *JNCI Cancer Spectrum.* doi:10.1093/jncics/pkz074

O'Toole, M.S., Renna, M.E., Mennin, D.S., & Fresco, D.M. (2019b). Changes in decentering and reappraisal temporally precede symptom reduction during emotion regulation therapy for generalized anxiety disorder with and without co-occurring depression. *Behavior Therapy, 56*, 1042–1052. doi:10.1016/j.beth.2018.12.005

Quintero, J.M., Mayville, E., Heimberg, R.G., Fresco, D.M., & Mennin, D.S. (in press). Implicit approach and avoidance motivational changes in GAD patients treated with emotion regulation therapy. *Journal of Behavioral and Cognitive Therapy.*

Raab, H.A., Sandman, C.F., Seeley, S., et al. (under review). Greater prefrontal recruitment associated with clinical improvement and regulatory skills in generalized anxiety patients following emotion regulation therapy: A pilot investigation.

Renna, M.E., Quintero, J.M., Fresco, D.M., & Mennin, D.S. (2017). Emotion regulation therapy: A mechanism-targeted treatment for disorders of distress. *Frontiers in Psychology, 8*, 98. doi:10.3389/fpsyg.2017.00098

Renna, M.E., Quintero, J.M., Soffer, A., Pino, M., Ader, L., Fresco, D.M., & Mennin, D.S. (2018a). A pilot study of emotion regulation therapy for generalized anxiety and depression: Findings from a diverse sample of young adults. *Behavior Therapy, 49*, 403–418.

Renna, M.E., Seeley, S.H., Heimberg, R.G., Etkin, A., Fresco, D.M., & Mennin, D.S. (2018b). Increased attention regulation from emotion regulation therapy for generalized anxiety disorder. *Cognitive Therapy and Research, 42*(2), 121–134.

Rheingold, A.A., Acierno, R., & Resnick, H.S. (2004). Trauma, posttraumatic stress disorder, and health risk behaviors. In P.P. Schnurr & B.L. Green (Eds.), *Trauma and health: Physical health consequences of exposure to extreme stress* (pp. 217–243). Washington, DC: American Psychological Association.

Ricard, M., & Browner, J. (2006). *Happiness: A guide to developing life's most important skill*. London, UK: Little, Brown.

Roemer, L., & Orsillo, S. (2009). *Guides to evidence-based treatment: Mindfulness- and acceptance-based behavioral therapies in practice*. New York: Guilford Press.

Salzberg, S. (1995). *Loving-kindness: The revolutionary art of happiness*. Boulder, CO: Shambhala.

Schut, A.J., Castonguay, L.G., & Borkovec, T.D. (2001). Compulsive checking behaviors in generalized anxiety disorder. *Journal of Clinical Psychology, 57*(6), 705–715.

Scult, M.A., Fresco, D.M., Gunning, F.M., Liston, C., Seeley, S.H., García, E., & Mennin, D.S. (2019). Changes in functional connectivity following treatment with emotion regulation therapy. *Frontiers in Behavioral Neuroscience, 13*, 10.

Seeley S.H., Etkin A., Liston C., Garcia E., Fresco, D.M., & Mennin, D.S. (in preparation). Decreased salience and frontoparietal regions activation in response to emotional conflict is associated with change in attention regulation in emotion regulation therapy for generalized anxiety disorder.

Segal, Z., Williams, J., & Teasdale, J. (2002). *Mindfulness-based cognitive therapy for depression*. New York: Guilford.

Skilton, M.R., Moulin, P., Terra, J.L., & Bonnet, F. (2007). Associations between anxiety, depression, and the metabolic syndrome. *Biological Psychiatry, 62*(11), 1251–1257. doi:10.1016/j.biopsych.2007.01.012

Steenkamp, M.M., Litz, B.T., Hoge, C.W., & Marmar, C.R. (2015). Psychotherapy for military-related PTSD: A review of randomized clinical trials. *JAMA, 314*(5), 489–500.

Strine, T.W., Mokdad, A.H., Dube, S.R., Balluz, L.S., Gonzalez, O., Berry, J.T.… Kroenke, K. (2008). The association of depression and anxiety with obesity and unhealthy behaviors among community-dwelling US adults. *General Hospital Psychiatry, 30*(2), 127–137. doi:10.1016/j.genhosppsych.2007.12.008

Tyrer, P., & Baldwin, D. (2006). Generalised anxiety disorder. *The Lancet, 368*(9553), 2156–2166. doi:10.1016/s0140-6736(06)69865-6

Watkins, E.R., Mullan, E., Wingrove, J., Rimes, K., Steiner, H., Bathurst, N.…Scott, J. (2011). Rumination-focused cognitive-behavioural therapy for residual depression: Phase II randomised controlled trial. *British Journal of Psychiatry, 199*(4), 317–322.

Wilson, K.G., & Murrell, A.R. (2004). Values work in acceptance and commitment therapy: Setting a course for behavioral treatment. In S.C. Hayes, V.M. Follette, & M. Linehan (Eds.), *Mindfulness and acceptance: Expanding the cognitive-behavioral tradition* (pp. 120–151). New York: Guilford Press.

Wolitzky-Taylor, K.B., Castriotta, N., Lenze, E.J., Stanley, M.A., & Craske, M.G. (2010). Anxiety disorders in older adults: A comprehensive review. *Depression and Anxiety, 27*(2), 190–211. doi:10.1002/da.20653

Zen, A.L., Whooley, M.A., Zhao, S., & Cohen, B.E. (2012). Post-traumatic stress disorder is associated with poor health behaviors: Findings from the heart and soul study. *Health Psychology, 31*(2), 194–201. doi:10.1037/a0025989

Chapter 5

Evidence-based psychotherapy – Rational Emotive Behavior Therapy and beyond

Problems, pitfalls, and promises in evaluating outcomes

Steven Jay Lynn, Craig P. Polizzi, Damla E. Aksen, and Fiona Sleight

We present Rational Emotive Behavior Therapy (REBT) as an example of a psychotherapy with a strong foundation of empirical support in the context of a broad discussion of the problems, pitfalls, and promises in evaluating treatment outcomes associated with REBT and other therapies. In contrast with pseudoscientific psychotherapy practices and those based on popular myths about psychotherapy, we argue that REBT can boast substantial empirical support in terms of favorable treatment outcomes and also in terms of the mediating role of irrational/dysfunctional beliefs as mechanisms that account for such outcomes. Further evaluation of REBT is called for in terms of theory and mechanisms of action, and in terms of extra-therapy or other explanatory variables, which can account for changes in functioning and symptoms over time. Evaluation frameworks that incorporate findings from well-controlled comparison trials that encompass diverse psychological conditions and samples, examine alternative interventions, and assess well-delineated components of multi-factorial treatments are a priority for a comprehensive evaluation of REBT. We conclude with a discussion of an emerging and welcome trend to develop and refine interventions, including REBT, that cross diagnostic and parochial therapy camps to ameliorate a variety of psychological conditions.

Over the past three decades, psychotherapy practitioners and consumers have welcomed a burgeoning movement toward evidence-based psychotherapy. Nevertheless, pseudoscientific therapies are still all too prevalent in the panoply of psychotherapies and often hold considerable appeal to the general public. In this chapter, we provide an overview of the vast landscape of pseudoscientific practices, the so-called scientist–practitioner gap, and the rise in scientific approaches to psychotherapy. We will consider Rational Emotive Behavior Therapy (REBT) as an example of a psychotherapy with a strong foundation of empirical support in the context of a broad discussion

DOI: 10.4324/9781003081593-7

of the problems, pitfalls, and promises in evaluating treatment outcomes associated with REBT and other therapies.

Albert Ellis (1994; see also Ellis, 1958) developed REBT as a variation of short-term Cognitive Behavioral Therapy (CBT) aimed at changing negative thinking patterns that contribute to distressing emotions and maladaptive behaviors. Hallmark elements of REBT include emphasis on enhancing unconditional self-acceptance and decreasing demanding beliefs (David et al., 2008). REBT is derived from Ellis's theoretical propositions that (1) cognitions can be identified and measured, (2) cognitions greatly contribute to human functioning and distress, and (3) irrational cognitions can be replaced with rational cognitions to produce adaptive psychosocial responses consistent with personal goals and values (David et al., 2010).

We will argue that REBT can boast substantial empirical support not only in terms of favorable treatment outcomes, but also in terms of the mediating role of irrational/dysfunctional beliefs as mechanisms that account for such outcomes. We will suggest that further evaluation of REBT in terms of theory and mechanisms of action, and in terms of extra-therapy or other explanatory variables, which can account for changes in functioning and symptoms over time, is necessary for a comprehensive evaluation of REBT. Finally, we will consider an emerging trend to develop and refine interventions that cross diagnostic and parochial therapy camps to ameliorate a variety of psychological conditions.

Myths and misconceptions of psychotherapy

Evaluating claims about psychotherapy is vitally important in guiding informed consumer decisions regarding treatments and in underscoring the value of psychotherapy (Gaudiano et al., 2016). Psychotherapy competes with pharmacotherapy and its use has decreased from 15.9% to 10.5% in mental health treatment settings (Olfson & Marcus, 2010). Nevertheless, psychotherapy is a frontline treatment that is more cost-effective than medications and better able to prevent relapse for anxiety and depression. Still, the image of psychotherapy is not altogether positive in the public eye due to stigma perpetuated by media, television, and movies, as myths and misconceptions about psychotherapy. The public and even some professional psychologists hold beliefs that potentially depreciate positive psychotherapy outcomes, are not supported by research, and are not typically accounted for in psychotherapy outcome studies (Lilienfeld et al., 2011).

For example, some individuals believe that deep personal exploration and insight are central to psychotherapy and individuals must be in therapy for many years to experience significant improvements. Emotional catharsis is also mistakenly believed to be a central element of psychotherapy.

In fact, catharsis absent positive cognitive restructuring of the meaning of the provoking situation can harm long-term adjustment (Littrell, 1998). Another misconception is that evidence-based, present-centered practices, such as REBT and cognitive behavior therapy (CBT), are not "real" therapy insofar as for a therapy to be successful it must confront the "root causes" of patient's psychological turmoil or risk symptom substitution or an untoward outcome. Participants who embrace this belief may engage in fruitless efforts to identify such causes and rectify past traumas or transgressions. Patients who believe falsely that they must engage with or "process" all painful emotions may "spend far more time wallowing in their feelings than attempting to restructure them constructively" (Lilienfeld et al., 2011, p. 313), as in REBT and CBT more generally.

These misconceptions can not only discourage people from consulting therapists, but also impede their engagement in psychotherapy and ability to maximize treatment gains. It is therefore important to (1) disabuse patients and the general public regarding misconceptions about psychotherapy and instill accurate, data-grounded beliefs and appropriate expectations and, more germane to our discussion, (2) assess whether accurate beliefs about psychotherapy or "rational beliefs," more generally, impact treatment gains (Macavei & McMahon, 2010). We suggest there exists a pressing need not only to evaluate and correct misconceptions, but also to (1) contrast evidence-based treatments sharply with less scientifically supported and pseudoscientific approaches and (2) design optimal schemes for evaluating psychotherapies and their mechanisms of action.

What is evidence-based practice?

Evidence-based practice is firmly grounded in the evaluation of psychotherapy outcomes. A perennial question regarding psychotherapy is: "What works best, for whom, and under what conditions?" Clinical scientists have made progress in addressing this question, but much work remains to be done. When conceptualizing evidence-based practice, psychologists commonly describe it in terms of a three-legged stool, where each leg is essential to provide support. The three legs are: clinical experience, clinical research, and patient preferences (Lilienfeld et al., 2014a). The goal of evidence-based practice is to provide clinicians with empirically validated methodologies to steer psychotherapy guided by evidence-based principles.

Lilienfeld and colleagues (2014a) identified five essential principles of evidence-based psychotherapy. First, effective psychological practice relies on an understanding of basic psychological science. Second, a humane approach to clinical practice is not inconsistent with science; it demands it. Third, clinical intuitions are important; the imperative is to be attuned to them, but not to embrace them uncritically. Fourth, high quality assessment is the bedrock of clinical work. Fifth, evaluation of psychotherapy is integral to amassing information regarding relatively new or understudied psychotherapies, to refining extant empirically supported approaches, and to deciding which interventions are most appropriate for treating diverse patients and disorders.

The primary reason why therapists might be reluctant to use evidence-based treatments is that they hold misconceptions about science-based practice. These misconceptions can include beliefs that evidence-based practice (1) stifles new treatments; (2) requires a "cookie cutter," one size fits all approach; (3) excludes nonspecific effects in therapy; (4) does not generalize to people not evaluated in controlled studies; (5) neglects evidence other than randomized controlled trials (RCTs); and (6) does not quantify therapeutic changes (Lilienfeld et al., 2014a). The belief that all treatments are equally effective may be the major hindrance to the utilization of evidence-based practice.

Unfortunately, many psychotherapists do not use well-established empirically supported methods. Approximately 83% reported that they never or rarely use prolonged exposure for posttraumatic stress disorder (Becker et al., 2004). Hipol and Deacon (2013) found that 73% of therapists reported not using therapist-guided exposure for obsessive compulsive disorder (OCD). Lilienfeld and colleagues (2011) documented that 21% and 44%, respectively, of practitioners who treat eating disorders administer CBT and interpersonal therapy either sometimes or never. Most therapists do not use empirically supported methods with clients with depression and panic attacks (Kessler et al., 2001).

Non-empirically supported methods are appealing for several reasons. Therapists sincerely want to help people, so they do what they think is right for their clients, absent a strong empirical or theoretical justification. Their treatments also give people hope, and therapists understandably desire a "quick fix" for their clients' problems. Therapists are also burdened with demanding schedules and are under pressure from insurance companies to document their treatment, so staying current with the extant literature is a "luxury." Finally, a lag exists between starting a new treatment and the rigorous evaluation of the intervention.

Taken together, these reasons point to a gulf between scientists and practitioners, which is often referred to as the scientist–practitioner gap. Ron Fox (2000), a former president of the American Psychological Association (APA), stated that "psychologists do not have to apologize for their treatments. Nor is there an actual need to prove their effectiveness," which reflects this scientist–practitioner gap (pp. 1–2). Consider also this statement from Healy (2002): "When treatments work, the condition being treated vanishes, and we don't need RCTs to see this happening" (p. 1). Yet, the conditions Healy (2002) is referring to may vanish for a plethora of reasons, which need to be accounted for in RCTs.

Can psychotherapy be evaluated?

Evaluation can be useful not only to ascertain the relative benefits of diverse psychotherapies and the contribution of particular treatment components to their overall success; evaluation can also be integrated into psychotherapy itself to steer therapist behavior, index the status of the therapeutic alliance, and determine how the client and the intervention are progressing. For example, brief questionnaires can be used in each psychotherapy session not only to track client progress but also to provide feedback to therapists and clients that can avert potential deterioration over sessions and negative outcomes (see Lambert, 2013).

Our discussion so far would suggest that psychotherapy can be evaluated. Although we strongly endorse this claim, it is not accepted universally. Of course, psychotherapies cannot be documented as empirically supported unless or until they are evaluated. Nevertheless, it is challenging to assess the more than 600 psychotherapies currently in vogue (Lilienfeld, 2007). Moreover, it can be daunting to evaluate psychotherapy due to the sheer number of potential variables that could conceivably impact psychotherapy outcome.

Corsini and Wedding (2008) were strong exponents of this position. In fact, they defended their decision not to include much scientific evidence bearing on the efficacy of each treatment featured in their widely used psychotherapy textbook on the following grounds. They cited Patterson (1987) approvingly, stating that, to subject psychotherapy to systematic research, "we would need (1) a taxonomy of client problems or psychological disorders...(2) a taxonomy of client personalities; (3) a taxonomy of therapeutic techniques...(4) a taxonomy of therapists; and (5) a taxonomy of circumstances. If we did have such a system of classification, the practical problems would be insurmountable. So, I conclude we don't need complex multivariate analyses and should abandon any attempt to do the crucial, perfect study of psychotherapy. It simply is not possible" (p. 247).

However, the fact that many variables, such as clients' personality traits and therapists' psychological characteristics, interact statistically in complex ways does not undermine the fact that some therapies are more effective overall relative to others, or demonstrate that the scientific method cannot rise to the challenge of evaluating diverse elements of psychotherapies. Thus, scientific evaluations of who seeks treatment, who benefits from it, and how therapist variables play a role are warranted, and we now consider some of the findings secured by such evaluations.

Lilienfeld et al. (2018) reviewed research relevant to who seeks treatment. Approximately 70% of people suffering from psychological conditions (e.g., anxiety, depression) do not have access to psychological services. Also, approximately 87% of uninsured children do not receive psychological services. Women more than men seek treatment, but both equally benefit.

African Americans and Hispanic Americans are less likely to seek services than Caucasian Americans. Ethnic minorities prefer therapists with similar backgrounds, but there is no consistent evidence suggesting that outcome is enhanced by ethnic or gender matches. Yet match may play a greater role when people are new to the culture. Accordingly, people can be helped by therapists who differ from them in significant ways, but who receives services depends, in part, on socioeconomic factors and cultural stigma. Unfortunately, studies that evaluate psychotherapies often do not consider socioeconomic and cultural variables, and these are not always matched across treatment conditions, even in randomized clinical trials (RCTs). Moreover, the influence of some variables might differ as a function of the psychotherapy employed such that therapist match might be more closely tied to positive outcomes in REBT, for example, than in other therapies such as behavior therapy.

Research on psychotherapies rarely considers the adjustment and mental health of the person prior to seeking psychotherapy, the situational context in which problems occur, and people's motivation for change. Nevertheless, some important findings have emerged: (1) Patient effects account for substantial variability in therapy outcome, but for minor differences within a specific disorder (Barth et al., 2013). (2) There are minimal differences in treatment response as a function of sex, age, depression, and medical disorders (Cuijpers et al., 2018). (3) The presence of anxiety or dysphoria motivates change (Frank, 1961, 1974; Miller et al, 1995). (4) People with situational or temporary problems often benefit from therapy (Gasperini et al., 1993; Steinmetz et al., 1983). (5) Finally, providing people with choice in the type of therapy they receive can enhance outcomes (Lindhiem et al., 2014).

The therapist also makes a difference in psychotherapy. Luborsky et al. (1986) found that therapist differences were stronger predictors of outcome than the treatments themselves, whereas Crits-Christoph and Mintz (1991) documented great variability in therapist effects across 27 studies, which accounted for 8.6% of variance in outcome. Although researchers have replicated therapist effects across different samples, findings regarding the strength of these effects vary among studies mostly likely due to variability in samples, outcome measures, and statistical analyses (Barkham et al., 2017).

Despite these mixed findings, the characteristics of effective therapists appear to be consistent across studies and modalities. These characteristics include verbal fluency, warmth, acceptance, empathy, affective regulation, focus on the client, and providing an explanation/rationale for a client's distress and a treatment plan (Castonguay & Hill, 2017). Effective therapists also engage in few negative communications with clients and reconcile with clients if a negative communication occurs by soliciting feedback and monitoring treatment. They are also flexible and roll with resistance by communicating hope and optimism (Constantino et al., 2012; Garske &

Anderson, 2003; Lilienfeld et al., 2018). These factors combined engender a strong working alliance that promotes therapeutic change (Wampold & Ulvenes, 2019). Although therapist choice may be as important as the choice of therapy, few studies have evaluated the interaction of treatments with therapist characteristics. Moreover, psychologists have advocated for personalized therapy that tailors interventions to the individuality of the patient (e.g., Norcross & Wampold, 2010). An APA task force, for example, suggested that therapy can be modified based on the client's reactance, preferences, culture, religion/spirituality, and expectations (see Norcross & Wampold, 2018).

Additionally, not all therapies have an equal evidence base. Many therapies are based on pseudoscience (i.e., beliefs and clinical practices mistakenly claimed to be or regarded to be based on or compatible with scientific method or empirically supported findings) and nonscience (i.e., nonempirically supported claims) (Lilienfeld et al., 2014a). Therapies based on pseudoscience and nonscience often make strong but unverified claims, which sets the stage for marketing countless interventions that promise far more than they deliver and render it difficult for consumers to distinguish these interventions from those with substantial empirical support. A smattering of these interventions includes neurolinguistic programming, thought field therapy, emotional freedom technique, facilitated communication, rage reduction therapy, sensory-motor integration therapy, rebirthing, reparenting, and holding therapy, to name a few.

In contrast, the promises of empirically supported psychotherapies are often based on psychological theories rigorously tested with controlled studies. For example, empirical studies have supported the theoretical framework of REBT. Cross-sectional and prospective studies have evidenced a positive association between dysphoric mood and irrational beliefs, especially demandingness, in individuals with depression and anxiety (e.g., Jackson et al., 2012; Nieuwenhuijsen et al., 2010; Szentágotai et al., 2008). REBT also holds that thinking patterns can create healthy (e.g., joy, appropriate anger) and unhealthy (e.g., fear, sadness, excessive anger) emotional reactions to events that are deemed imperative to be experienced fully to facilitate recovery (Ellis et al., 2010). This therapeutic process is consistent with research indicating that engagement with affective states is critical in treating psychiatric conditions (e.g., Bach & Hayes, 2002; Lynn et al., 2006; Mellinger & Lynn, 2003). Accordingly, REBT may be a particularly cost-effective treatment because it efficiently and effectively disrupts dysfunctional autobiographical beliefs and promotes emotional engagement (Sava et al., 2008). Indeed, researchers have reported treatment gains across multiple conditions ranging from schizophrenia to posttraumatic stress disorder (Hyland et al., 2015; Kingdon & Turkington, 2006), as well as other conditions discussed below.

A challenge for evaluation: can change be attributed to the psychotherapy administered?

Specific effects of psychotherapy are those related to techniques associated with the protocols of a treatment modality (e.g., REBT, psychodynamic, interpersonal) that are believed or found to be associated with the effectiveness or efficacy of the treatment (Lohr et al., 2003). Specific factors can account for nontrivial differences in treatment outcomes, especially in anxiety disorders (Tolin, 2014) and obsessive-compulsive disorder (Strauss et al., 2018). In contrast, nonspecific effects based on common factors that exist across therapies, which include positive expectations, the therapeutic relationship (empathy, alliance, and affirmation), goal elaboration (agreement on tasks and actions), a healing setting, provision of a therapy rationale, practice of new behaviors, provision of a new perspective, interpersonal learning, and therapist effects, can also exert a strong effect on therapeutic change (Wampold & Ulvenes, 2019). Although not all psychotherapies are equal in effectiveness for all conditions, there typically are not vast differences, if any, among well-established interventions. Thus, nonspecific and specific effects both matter, and therapists would do well to eschew "either–or" thinking. Nevertheless, a critical empirical challenge is to disentangle nonspecific and specific effects in treatment and experimental contexts.

A prominent challenge in evaluating psychotherapies is that people may improve for various reasons apart from the specific factors associated with a particular treatment. As such, even pseudoscientific therapies may show treatment gains. More specifically, Lilienfeld and colleagues (2014b) identified reasons why people experience apparent benefits from therapy that have little or nothing to do with the treatment implemented. These reasons need to be considered in evaluating psychotherapies to isolate any specific effects of REBT. The placebo effect (i.e., the beneficial effect produced by a medication or treatment due to positive belief in the effectiveness of the intervention) is approximately 80% as effective as antidepressant medication in treating depression (Kirsch et al., 2002). Illusory placebo effects occur when people believe conditions improve in the absence of actual change in outcome measures (e.g., subliminal audiotapes with "wrong" message/self-esteem-enhanced memory). The novelty effect (i.e., excitement about a new intervention) also impacts treatment outcome; approximately 15% of patients improve between the initial phone call and the first psychotherapy session (Howard et al., 1986). Additionally, spontaneous remission (i.e., unplanned or unexpected symptom reductions) estimates range from 15% to 70% in psychotherapy (see Lilienfeld et al., 2014b).

The cyclical nature of many disorders (e.g., bipolar disorder, cyclothymic disorder) may also contribute to perceived improvements in psychotherapy. Regression to the mean can occur in psychotherapy studies because most patients initiate therapy when they are most symptomatic and improve even in the absence of treatment. Positive life events outside therapy, including improved family dynamics, exercise, medical treatment, can also exert positive effects mistaken for treatment effects. Moreover, demand characteristics also may enhance treatment outcome and bias self-reports of improvement. Individuals may be misdiagnosed at the start of treatment; when the diagnosis is clarified, it may not be as severe as the initial diagnosis. Unfortunately, many of these variables and others (Lilienfeld et al., 2014b) are rarely accounted for statistically or in terms of measures administered in research on REBT and other psychotherapies. Nevertheless, some REBT studies include attention-placebo comparison conditions to control for expectancies and other non-specific effects (e.g., Iftene et al., 2015; Sava et al., 2008).

What is considered evidence-based: "a moving target"

What is considered evidence-based varies considerably among researchers, classification schemes, and international organizations. Evaluative frameworks generate conflicting standards, which engenders confusion based on different guidelines from the National Institute of Health (NIH) versus APA Division 12 versus the American Psychiatric Association versus the National Institute for Health and Care Excellence (NICE), for example. Moreover, none of these frameworks considers support or lack of it for theory or claimed therapeutic mechanisms (David & Montgomery, 2011; David et al., 2018). Under these circumstances, a therapy based on voodoo practices could be considered empirically supported if it produced better outcomes relative to a waitlist control condition.

Clearly, a specific and comprehensive evaluative framework is needed to optimize future outcome studies of REBT. David and Montgomery (2011; see also David et al., 2018) proposed such a framework that evaluates the theory that undergirds a treatment independent of evaluation of the treatment package (e.g., methods, techniques). To be categorized as a well-supported treatment package, it must be empirically supported by at least two carefully conducted RCTs. A theory is deemed to be well-supported based on (1) experimental studies and/or (2) analyses of treatment components, client–treatment interactions, and/or mediation/moderation analyses in well-controlled clinical trials. Theories and treatments can be deemed supported by equivocal evidence when they are based on studies not involving empirical data or studies that provided preliminary or mixed data (supporting and nonsupporting evidence). Theories and treatments are categorized as based on strong contradictory evidence when they are not empirically supported in at least two rigorous RCTs conducted by two independent investigators or research teams.

The APA (2016) has identified REBT as having modest empirical support, and NICE (2009) included REBT in its guidelines for evidence-based practice for depression. Early meta-analytic studies supported REBT as an empirically supported form of CBT and as an efficacious psychotherapy (e.g., Engels et al.,1993; Lyons & Woods, 1991). In a later RCT, David and colleagues (2008) found that REBT is as efficient as cognitive therapy and medication at reducing depressive mood and thinking post-treatment and more efficient than medication at six-month follow-up. Changes in irrational beliefs were related to changes in depressed mood and thinking. More recent RCTs have found that REBT elicits decreased depression, negative beliefs, and physical pain compared with no intervention comparison conditions (e.g., Mahigir et al., 2012; Ogbuanya et al., 2018; Onuigbo et al., 2019; Zhaleh et al., 2014). Additionally, RCTs indicated REBT produced greater increases in self-efficacy and well-being compared with a no intervention control condition (Jalali et al., 2014; Kim et al., 2015). Another RCT involving REBT, pharmacotherapy, and their combination documented that all treatments yielded reductions on subjective, cognitive, and biological measures of depression in youths with major depressive disorder (Iftene et al., 2015). REBT was also effective in reducing negative thinking patterns in controlled trials with athlete samples (e.g., Cunningham & Turner, 2016; Turner et al., 2014; Turner et al., 2020).

Researchers have suggested that REBT alleviates psychophysiological symptoms and distress related to chronic medical conditions. Individuals with Type-2 diabetes treated with REBT experienced greater reductions in depression compared with individuals who received standard counseling (Eseadi et al., 2017). REBT has also proved effective in reducing mild hypertension at two-month follow-up (Drazen et al., 1982) and decreased preoccupation with asthma symptoms and emotional distress (Maes & Schlosser, 1988). Interventions that combined REBT with hypnosis were found to decrease fatigue in breast cancer radiotherapy patients over the entire course of treatment (Montgomery et al., 2009). David et al. (2018) classified REBT as a category III theory-driven psychotherapy with strong supporting evidence for its etiological theory of depression but with preliminary data supporting its efficacy relative to other treatments (e.g., correlational studies, few RCTs).

Findings are mixed with respect to the superiority of REBT over other empirically supported treatments. A RCT of major depressive disorder found that changes in depressive symptoms, depression-free days, and quality of life did not differ across REBT, cognitive therapy, and Prozac treatment (Sava et al., 2008). Dialectical Behavior Therapy (DBT) may be more efficient than REBT at addressing irrational thinking because DBT exerts a broader impact on irrational beliefs compared with REBT, which focuses on a narrower range of beliefs (Asmand et al., 2015). Future RCTs are necessary to (1) establish REBT's effectiveness compared with other evidence-based psychotherapies; (2) test if irrational beliefs mediate and/or moderate REBT treatment outcomes, especially decreased depression; and

(3) determine the role of irrational beliefs across various manifestations of psychopathology.

Future directions and conclusions

Despite certain criticisms, considerable empirical support exists for REBT, which has shown promise in ameliorating many conditions. Future evaluation schemes should consider or control for: (1) co-existing conditions, (2) medication or medication compliance, (3) socioeconomic status and cultural variables, and (4) prior treatments. The weight of evidence in terms of strong (e.g., placebo pill, treatment-as-usual) versus weak (e.g., waitlist control) comparison conditions should be considered as well (Cuijpers et al., 2018; David et al., 2018). To maximize internal and external validity, we suggest future studies evaluate variables of interest (e.g., patient, therapist effects) across individual (e.g., therapist, client personality characteristics), naturalistic (e.g., community, independent practice settings), experimental (e.g., manipulating rapport), and process (e.g., within/ between treatment sessions) analyses and across short- and long-term interventions, accounting for spontaneous remission.

Future schemes should incorporate meta-analytic studies that include risk of bias assessments and report treatment effect sizes. Internet delivery of psychotherapy is another promising area in studies of REBT. Therapy process studies that examine therapist–patient interactions may also prove valuable for future schemes. Personalized versus nonpersonalized approaches can be studied to determine which treatments are more effective based on the condition treated. REBT could be presented across different modalities and levels of personalization to ascertain optimum delivery for adults, university students, or individuals with comorbid conditions as well as determine the comparability of treatment as usual with Internet-delivered treatment or teletherapy.

No systematic research, to our knowledge, exists that evaluates REBT in terms of the Research Domain Criteria (RDoC) developed by the National Institute of Mental Health (Insel et al., 2010). RDoC is a broad framework that consists of multiple dimensions for studying psychiatric disorders and encompasses genetics, neuroscience, and social interactions. For example, researchers can evaluate depression in terms of dysfunction in brain circuits related to reward processing and dopamine, supplemented with genetic and psychosocial data. RDoC could assay how REBT impacts different biopsychosocial processes across multiple dimensions of psychological disorders and dysfunctions.

Researchers informed by novel evaluation schemes can consider how therapy is conducted in the "real world." Many clinical practitioners implement overlapping therapy techniques and blend techniques from different schools of therapy. Future schemes can incorporate research on how to best combine modalities, such as REBT and Acceptance and Commitment Therapy (ACT) and exposure therapy. Also, many clients seek therapy to address quality of life problems beyond symptoms of depression or anxiety, for example. More complex and nuanced schemes can consider the extent to which interventions enhance quality of life among people with different personality characteristics. Measuring changes in cognition, affect, and behavior in the naturalistic environment with cell phones and other recording devices and assessing adaptive and maladaptive patterns of sleep via actigraphy devices and increasingly sophisticated fitness watch programs can address concerns about the ecological validity of assessment and the transfer of treatment gains to everyday life beyond retrospective patient self-reports.

The nascent movement toward transdiagnostic and transtheoretical therapies extends beyond treating a narrow group of symptoms within the purview of specific schools of therapy to target change principles common across diverse emotional disorders. We suggest that cognitive-behavioral-affective mechanisms associated with REBT are likely to be effective across many psychological disorders and conditions yet can be targeted to irrational beliefs associated with different disorders such as depression. Moreover, the modular nature of some transdiagnostic and transtheoretical therapies permits evaluation of the effectiveness of discrete components as well as the entire protocol, setting the stage for refining and tailoring interventions to address specific needs. Barlow's (Barlow et al., 2020) empirically supported unified protocol (UP) for treating emotional disorders, for example, focuses on rapport building, psychoeducation, enhancing motivation and expectancy, awareness of emotions and sensations, cognitive reappraisal, nonavoidance (i.e., exposure, mindfulness), and relapse prevention. Many of these components are embedded in REBT. The UP has proved effective in treating anxiety, depression, eating disorders, sexual dysfunctions, bipolar disorder, and dissociative disorders (Barlow et al., 2020; Mohajerin et al., 2019).

In conclusion, REBT exemplifies the value of psychotherapy evaluation. Sophisticated and empirically based schemes are imperative to understanding how specific and well-described interventions are more or less effective in treating diverse conditions and in identifying combinations of modalities to optimize and personalize outcomes. Information from these schemes can potentially be used to enhance REBT and create more refined REBT-informed transdiagnostic/transtheoretical interventions that enhance treatment gains.

References

American Psychological Association (APA). (2016). *Psychological Treatments*. Retrieved 06/10/21 from www.div12.org/treatments/

Asmand, P., Mami, S., & Valizadeh, R. (2015). The effectiveness of dialectical behavior therapy and rational emotive behavior therapy in irrational believes treatment among young male prisoners who have antisocial personality disorder in Ilam Prison. *International Journal of Health System and Disaster Management*, *3*(2), 68–73. https://doi.org/10.4103/2347-9019.147135

Bach, P., & Hayes, S.C. (2002). The use of acceptance and commitment therapy to prevent the rehospitalization of psychotic patients: A randomized controlled trial. *Journal of Consulting and Clinical Psychology*, *70*(5), 1129–1139. https://doi.org/10.1037/0022-006X.70.5.1129

Barkham, M., Lutz, W., Lambert, M.J., & Saxon, D. (2017). Therapist effects, effective therapists, and the law of variability. In L.G. Castonguay & C.E. Hill (Eds.), *How and why are some therapists better than others? Understanding therapist effects* (pp. 13–36). Washington, DC: American Psychological Association. https://doi.org/10.1037/0000034-002

Barlow, D.H., Harris, B.A., Eustis, E.H., & Farchione, T.J. (2020). The unified protocol for transdiagnostic treatment of emotional disorders. *World Psychiatry: Official Journal of the World Psychiatric Association (WPA)*, *19*(2), 245–246. https://doi.org/10.1002/wps.20748

Barth, J., Munder, T., Gerger, H., Nuesch, E., Trelle, S., Znoj, H., Juni, P., & Cuijpers P. (2013). Comparative efficacy of seven psychotherapeutic interventions for patients with depression: A network meta-analysis. *PLoS Medicine*, *10*(5). https://doi.org/10.1371/journal.pmed.1001454

Becker, C.B., Zayfert, C., & Anderson, E. (2004). A survey of psychologists' attitudes towards and utilization of exposure therapy for PTSD. *Behavior Research and Therapy*, *42*(3), 277–292. https://doi.org/10.1016/S0005-7967(03)00138-4

Castonguay, L.G., & Hill, C.E. (Eds.). (2017). *How and why are some therapists better than others? Understanding therapist effects*. Washington, DC: American Psychological Association.

Constantino, M.J., Ametrano, R.M., & Greenberg, R.P. (2012). Clinician interventions and participant characteristics that foster adaptive patient expectations for psychotherapy and psychotherapeutic change. *Psychotherapy*, *49*(4), 557–569. https://doi.org/10.1037/a0029440

Corsini, R.J., & Wedding, D. (Eds.). (2008). *Current Psychotherapies*. Belmont, CA: Thomson Higher Education.

Crits-Christoph, P., & Mintz, J. (1991). Implications of therapist effects for the design and analysis of comparative studies of psychotherapies. *Journal of Consulting and Clinical Psychology*, *59*(1), 20–26. https://doi.org/10.1037/0022-006X.59.1.20

Cuijpers, P., Karyotaki, E., Reijnders, M., & Huibers, M.J.H. (2018). Who benefits from psychotherapies for adult depression? A meta-analytic update of the evidence. *Cognitive Behaviour Therapy*, *47*(2), 91–106. https://doi.org/10.1080/16506073.2017.1420098

Cunningham, R., & Turner, M.J. (2016). Using Rational Emotive Behavior Therapy (REBT) with Mixed Martial Arts (MMA) athletes to reduce irrational beliefs and increase unconditional self-acceptance. *Journal of Rational-Emotive & Cognitive-Behavior Therapy*, *34*(4), 289–309. https://doi.org/10.1007/s10942-016-0240-4

David, D., & Montgomery G.H. (2011). The scientific status of psychotherapies: A new evaluative framework for evidence-based psychosocial interventions. *Clinical Psychology: Science and Practice*, *18*(2), 89–99. https://doi.org/10.1111/j.1468-2850.2011.01239.x

David, D., Lynn, S.J., & Ellis, A. (Eds.). (2010). *Rational and irrational beliefs: Research, theory, and clinical practice.* New York: Oxford University Press.

David, D., Lynn, S.J., & Montgomery, G.H. (Eds.). (2018). *Evidence-based psychotherapy: The state of the science and practice.* Hoboken, NJ: Wiley-Blackwell.

David, D., Szentágotai, A., Lupu, V., & Cosman, D. (2008). Rational emotive behavior therapy, cognitive therapy, and medication in the treatment of major depressive disorder: A randomized clinical trial, posttreatment outcomes, and six-month follow-up. *Journal of Clinical Psychology*, *64*(6), 728–746. https://doi.org/10.1002/jclp.20487

Drazen, M., Nevid, J.S., Pace, N., & O'Brien, R.M. (1982). Worksite-based behavioral treatment of mild hypertension. *Journal of Occupational Medicine*, *24*(7), 511–514.

Ellis, A. (1958). Rational psychotherapy. *Journal of General Psychology*, *59*, 35–49.

Ellis, A. (1994). *Reason and emotion in psychotherapy: A comprehensive method of treating human disturbances. Revised and updated.* Secaucus, NJ: Carol.

Ellis, A., David, D., & Lynn, S.J. (2010). *Rational and irrational beliefs: A historical and conceptual perspective.* In D. David, S.J. Lynn, & A. Ellis (Eds.), *Rational and irrational beliefs: Research, theory, and clinical practice* (pp. 3–22). New York: Oxford University Press.

Engels, G.I., Garnefski, N., & Diekstra, R.F. (1993). Efficacy of rational-emotive therapy: A quantitative analysis. *Journal of Consulting and Clinical Psychology*, *61*(6), 1083–1090. https://doi.org/10.1037/0022-006X.61.6.1083

Eseadi, C., Onwuka, G.T., Otu, M.S., Umoke, P.C., Onyechi, K.C., Okere, A.U., & Edeh, N.C. (2017). Effects of rational emotive cognitive behavioral coaching on depression among Type 2 diabetic inpatients. *Journal of Rational-Emotive & Cognitive-Behavior Therapy*, *35*(4), 363–382. https://doi.org/10.1007/s10942-017-0266-2

Fox, R.E. (2000). The dark side of evidence-based treatment. *Practitioner Focus* [APA Practice Directorate newsletter]. Retrieved 06/07/20 from www.apa.org/practice/pf/jan00/capp chair.html

Frank, J.D. (1961). *Persuasion and healing: A comparative study of psychotherapy.* Baltimore, MD: Johns Hopkins University Press.

Frank, J.D. (1974). Psychotherapy: The restoration of morale. *American Journal of Psychiatry*, *131*(3), 271–274. https://doi.org/10.1176/ajp.131.3.271

Garske, J.P., & Anderson, T. (2003). *Toward a science of psychotherapy research: Present status and evaluation.* In S.O. Lilienfeld, S.J. Lynn, & J.M. Lohr (Eds.), *Science and pseudoscience in clinical psychology* (pp. 145–175). New York: Guilford Press.

Gasperini, M., Scherillo, P., Manfredonia, M.G., Franchini L., & Smeraldi E. (1993). A study of relapses in subjects with mood disorder on lithium treatment. *European Neuropsychopharmacology: The Journal of the European College of Neuropsychopharmacology*, *3*(2), 103–110. https://doi.org/10.1016/0924-977x(93)90261-j

Gaudiano, B.A., Ellenberg, S.R., Schofield, C.A., & Rifkin, L.S. (2016). A randomized survey of the public's expectancies and willingness to participate in clinical trials of antidepressants versus psychotherapy for depression. *Primary Care Companion for CNS Disorders, 18*(1). https://doi.org/10.4088/PCC.15m01879

Healy, D. (2002). *Randomized controlled trials: Evidence based psychiatry.* Retrieved from www.ahrp.org/COI/healy0802.php

Hipol, L.J., & Deacon, B.J. (2013). Dissemination of evidence-based practices for anxiety disorders in Wyoming: A survey of practicing psychotherapists. *Behavior Modification, 37*(2), 170–188. https://doi.org/10.1177/0145445512458794

Howard, K.I., Kopta, S.M., Krause, M.S., & Orlinsky D.E. (1986). The dose–effect relationship in psychotherapy. *American Psychologist, 41*(2), 159–164. https://doi.org/10.1037/0003-066X.41.2.159

Hyland, P., Shevlin, M., Adamson, G., & Boduszek, D. (2015). Irrational beliefs in posttraumatic stress responses: A rational emotive behavior therapy approach. *Journal of Loss and Trauma, 20*(2), 171–188. https://doi.org/10.1080/15325024.2013.839772

Iftene, F., Predescu, E., Stefan, S., & David, D. (2015). Rational-emotive and cognitive-behavior therapy (REBT/CBT) versus pharmacotherapy versus REBT/CBT plus pharmacotherapy in the treatment of major depressive disorder in youth: A randomized clinical trial. *Psychiatry Research, 225*(3), 687–694. https://doi.org/10.1016/j.psychres.2014.11.021

Insel, T., Cuthbert, B., Garvey, M., Heinssen, R., Pine, D.S., Quinn, K., Sanislow, C., & Wang, P. (2010). Research domain criteria (RDoC): Toward a new classification framework for research on mental disorders. *American Journal of Psychiatry, 167*(7), 748–751. https://doi.org/10.1176/appi.ajp.2010.09091379

Jackson, C.J., Izadikah, Z., & Oei, T.P. (2012). Mechanisms underlying REBT in mood disordered patients: Predicting depression from the hybrid model of learning. *Journal of Affective Disorders, 139*(1), 30–39. https://doi.org/10.1016/j.jad.2011.09.025

Jalali, M.D.M., Moussavi, M.S., Yazdi, S.A.A., & Fadardi, J.S. (2014). Effectiveness of rational emotive behavior therapy on psychological well-being of people with late blindness. *Journal of Rational-Emotive & Cognitive-Behavior Therapy, 32*, 233–247. https://doi.org/10.1007/s10942-014-0191-6

Kessler, R.C., Soukup, J., Davis, R.B., Foster, D.F., Wilkey, S.A., Van Rompay, M.I., & Eisenberg, D.M. (2001). The use of complementary and alternative therapies to treat anxiety and depression in the United States. *American Journal of Psychiatry, 158*(2), 289–294. https://doi.org/10.1176/appi.ajp.158.2.289

Kim, M.A., Kim, J., & Kim, E.J. (2015). Effects of rational emotive behavior therapy for senior nursing students on coping strategies and self-efficacy. *Nurse Education Today, 35*(3), 456–460. https://doi.org/10.1016/j.nedt.2014.11.013

Kingdon, D., & Turkington, D. (2006). The ABCs of cognitive-behavioral therapy for schizophrenia. *Psychiatric Times, 23*(7), 49–50.

Kirsch, I., Moore, T.J., Scoboria, A., & Nicholls, S.S. (2002). The emperor's new drugs: An analysis of antidepressant medication data submitted to the US Food and Drug Administration. *Prevention & Treatment, 5*(1), 23. https://doi.org/10.1037/1522-3736.5.1.523a

Lambert, M.J. (2013). *Bergin and Garfield's handbook of psychotherapy and behavior change* (6th ed.). Hoboken, NJ: John Wiley & Sons.

Lilienfeld, S.O. (2007). Psychological treatments that cause harm. *Perspectives on Psychological Science, 2*(1), 53–70. https://doi.org/10.1111/j.1745-6916.2007.00029.x

Lilienfeld, S.O., Lynn, S.J., & Lohr, J. (2014a). Science and pseudoscience in clinical psychology. New York: Guilford Press.

Lilienfeld, S.O., Lynn, S.J., & Namy, L. (2018). *Psychology: From inquiry to understanding* (5th ed.). London, UK: Pearson Higher Education AU.

Lilienfeld, S.O., Lynn, S.J., Ruscio, J., & Beyerstein, B.L. (2011). *50 great myths of popular psychology: Shattering widespread misconceptions about human behavior.* Hoboken, NJ: John Wiley & Sons.

Lilienfeld, S.O., Ritschel, L.A., Lynn, S.J., Cautin, R.L., & Latzman, R.D. (2014b). Why ineffective psychotherapies appear to work: A taxonomy of causes of spurious therapeutic effectiveness. *Perspectives on Psychological Science, 9*(4), 355–387. https://doi.org/10.1177/1745691614535216

Lindhiem, O., Bennett, C.B., Trentacosta, C.J., & McLear, C. (2014). Client preferences affect treatment satisfaction, completion, and clinical outcome: A meta-analysis. *Clinical Psychology Review, 34*(6), 506–517. https://doi.org/10.1016/j.cpr.2014.06.002

Littrell, J. (1998). Is the reexperience of painful emotion therapeutic? *Clinical Psychology Review, 18*(1), 71–102. https://doi.org/10.1016/S0272-7358(97)00046-9

Lohr, J.M., DeMaio, C., & McGlynn, F.D. (2003). Specific and nonspecific treatment factors in the experimental analysis of behavioral treatment efficacy. *Behavior Modification, 27*(3), 322–368. https://doi.org/10.1177/0145445503027003005

Luborsky, L., Crits-Christoph, P., McLellan, A.T., Woody, G., Piper, W., Liberman, B., Imber, S., & Pilkonis, P. (1986). Do therapists vary much in their success? Findings from four outcome studies. *American Journal of Orthopsychiatry, 56*(4), 501–512. https://doi.org/10.1111/j.1939-0025.1986.tb03483.x

Lynn, S.J., Das, L.S., Hallquist, M.N., & Williams, J.C. (2006). Mindfulness, acceptance, and hypnosis: Cognitive and clinical perspectives. *International Journal of Clinical and Experimental Hypnosis, 54*(2), 143–166. https://doi.org/10.1080/00207140500528240

Lyons, L.C., & Woods, P.J. (1991). The efficacy of rational-emotive therapy: A quantitative review of the outcome research. *Clinical Psychology Review, 11*(4), 357–369. https://doi.org/10.1016/0272-7358(91)90113-9

Macavei, B., & McMahon, J. (2010). The assessment of rational and irrational beliefs. In D. David, S.J. Lynn, & A. Ellis (Eds.), *Rational and irrational beliefs: Research, theory and clinical practice* (pp. 115–132). New York: Oxford University Press.

Maes, S., & Schlosser, M. (1988). Changing health behaviour outcomes in asthmatic patients: A pilot intervention study. *Social Science & Medicine, 26*(3), 359–364. https://doi.org/10.1016/0277-9536(88)90401-7

Mahigir, F., Khanehkeshi, A., & Karimi, A. (2012). Psychological treatment for pain among cancer patients by rational-emotive behavior therapy: Efficacy in both India and Iran. *Asian Pacific Journal of Cancer Prevention, 13*(9), 4561–4565. https://doi.org/10.7314/apjcp.2012.13.9.4561

Mellinger, D.I., & Lynn, S.J. (2003). *The monster in the cave: How to face your fears and anxieties and live your life.* New York: Berkley/Putnam-Penguin.

Miller, J.J., Fletcher, K., & Kabat-Zinn, J. (1995). Three-year follow-up and clinical implications of a mindfulness meditation-based stress reduction intervention in the treatment of anxiety disorders. *General Hospital Psychiatry, 17,* 192–200.

Mohajerin, B., Lynn, S.J., Bakhtiyari, M., & Dolatshah, B. (2019). Evaluating the unified protocol in the treatment of dissociative identity disorder. *Cognitive and Behavioral Practice.* https://doi.org/10.1016/j.cbpra.2019.07.012

Montgomery, G.H., Kangas, M., David, D., Hallquist, M.N., Green, S., Bovbjerg, D.H., & Schnur, J.B. (2009). Fatigue during breast cancer radiotherapy: An initial randomized study of cognitive-behavioral therapy plus hypnosis. *Health Psychology, 28*(3), 317–322. https://doi.org/10.1037/a0013582

National Institute for Health and Care Excellence. (2009). *Treatment and management of depression in adults, including adults with a chronic physical health problem.* London, UK: National Institute for Health and Care Excellence.

Nieuwenhuijsen, K., Verbeek, J.H., de Boer, A.G., Blonk, R.W., & van Dijk, F.J. (2010). Irrational beliefs in employees with an adjustment, a depressive, or an anxiety disorder: A prospective cohort study. *Journal of Rational-Emotive & Cognitive-Behavior Therapy, 28*(2), 57–72. https://doi.org/10.1007/s10942-007-0075-0

Norcross, J.C., & Wampold, B.E. (2010). What works for whom: Tailoring psychotherapy to the person. *Journal of Clinical Psychology, 67*(2), 127–132. https://doi.org/10.1002/jclp.20764

Norcross, J.C., & Wampold, B.E. (2018). A new therapy for each patient: Evidence-based relationships and responsiveness. *Journal of Clinical Psychology, 74*(11), 1889–1906.

Ogbuanya, T.C., Eseadi, C., Orji, C.T., Anyanwu, J.I., Ede, M.O., & Bakare, J. (2018). Effect of rational emotive behavior therapy on negative career thoughts of students in technical colleges in Nigeria. *Psychological Reports, 121*(2), 356–374. https://doi.org/10.1177/0033294117724449

Olfson, M., & Marcus, S.C. (2010). National trends in outpatient psychotherapy. *American Journal of Psychiatry, 167*(12), 1456–1463. https://doi.org/10.1176/appi.ajp.2010.10040570

Onuigbo, L.N., Eseadi, C., Ebifa, S., Ugwu, U.C., Onyishi, C.N., & Oyeoku, E.K. (2019). Effect of rational emotive behavior therapy program on depressive symptoms among university students with blindness in Nigeria. *Journal of Rational-Emotive & Cognitive-Behavior Therapy, 37,* 17–38. https://doi.org/10.1007/s10942-018-0297-3

Patterson, C.H. (1987). Comments. *Person-Centered Review, 1,* 246–248.

Sava, F.A., Yates, B.T., Lupu, V., Szentágotai, A., & David, D. (2008). Cost-effectiveness and cost-utility of cognitive therapy, rational emotive behavioral therapy, and fluoxetine (Prozac) in treating depression: A randomized clinical trial. *Journal of Clinical Psychology, 65*(1), 36–52. https://doi.org/10.1002/jclp.20550

Steinmetz, J.L., Lewinsohn, P.M., & Antonucci, D.O. (1983). Prediction of individual outcome in a group intervention for depression. *Journal of Consulting and Clinical Psychology, 51*(3), 331–337. https://doi.org/10.1037/0022-006X.51.3.331

Strauss, A.Y., Huppert, J.D., Simpson, H.B., & Foa, E.B. (2018). What matters more? Common or specific factors in cognitive behavioral therapy for OCD: Therapeutic alliance and expectations as predictors of treatment outcome. *Behaviour Research and Therapy, 105,* 43–51. https://doi.org/10.1016/j.brat.2018.03.007

Szentágotai, A., David, D., Lupu, V., & Cosman, D. (2008). Rational emotive therapy, cognitive therapy and medication in the treatment of major depressive disorder: Theory of change analysis. *Psychotherapy: Theory, Research, Practice, Training, 45*(4), 523–538.

Tolin, D.F. (2014). Beating a dead dodo bird: Looking at signal vs. noise in cognitive- behavioral therapy for anxiety disorders. *Clinical Psychology: Science and Practice, 21*(4), 351–362. https://doi.org/10.1111/cpsp.12080

Turner, M.J., Ewen, D., & Barker, J.B. (2020). An idiographic single-case study examining the use of rational emotive behavior therapy (REBT) with three amateur golfers to alleviate social anxiety. *Journal of Applied Sport Psychology, 32*(2), 186–204. https://doi.org/10.1080/10413200.2018.1496186

Turner, M.J., Slater, M.J., & Barker, J.B. (2014). Not the end of the world: The effects of rational-emotive behavior therapy (REBT) on irrational beliefs in elite soccer academy athletes. *Journal of Applied Sport Psychology, 26*(2), 144–156. https://doi.org/10.1080/10413200.2013.812159

Wampold, B.E., & Ulvenes, P.G. (2019). Integration of common factors and specific ingredients. In J.C. Norcross & M.R. Goldfried (Eds.), *Handbook of psychotherapy integration* (3rd ed., pp. 69–87). New York: Oxford University Press.

Zhaleh, N., Zarbakhsh, M., & Faramarzi, M. (2014). Effectiveness of rational-emotive behavior therapy on the level of depression among female adolescents. *Journal of Applied Environmental and Biological Sciences, 4*(4), 102–107.

Chapter 6

Avoiding pitfalls in clinical trials and meta-analyses of REBT and other psychotherapies

Irving Kirsch

This chapter discusses some often-ignored problems in clinical research and meta-analyses and proposes the four reforms that can overcome those problems: 1. Avoid dichotomizing continuous variables, a frequent practice that has been widely condemned by statisticians as equivalent to discarding one third or more of the data. 2. To avoid the "efficacy paradox," analyze within-group differences as well as between-group differences. 3. To facilitate subsequent meta-analysis, report exact means of and standard deviations of baseline, endpoint, and difference scores in all clinical trials. 4. Do not attempt to construct sham treatments to control for the placebo effect in psychotherapy, because adequate placebo psychotherapies are impossible to construct, and the factors underlying the placebo effect (e.g., expectancy change) are among the specific active ingredients of effective psychotherapy.

One of the strengths of cognitive behavioral psychotherapies, of which rational emotive behavior therapy (REBT) was the first, is their commitment to research on the efficacy and mechanisms of treatment. However, it is important that psychotherapy research be well designed and executed. Much has been written about design problems in clinical trials generally, including such issues as publication bias, failures of replication, problems with blinding, etc. Here I address some often-ignored problems that can easily be remedied when designing clinical trials and meta-analyses of those trials. Some of these problems and solutions can be applied to psychological and medical research in general. Others are specific to psychotherapy.

Do not dichotomize continuous variables

Some outcomes are naturally dichotomous (e.g., pregnancy and death). Others are continuous (e.g., pain, depression, and anxiety). It is a common practice in medical and psychological research to dichotomize continuous variables. For example, participants may be categorized as responders/non-responders, remitters/non-remitters, young/old, mild/severe, etc. The statistical pitfalls of dichotomization have been well documented (Altman & Royston, 2006; Cohen, 1983; MacCallum, Zhang, Preacher, & Rucker,

DOI: 10.4324/9781003081593-8

2002; Royston, Altman, & Sauerbrei, 2006; Streiner, 2002). As described by Jacob Cohen in 1983, dichotomization of continuous data results in a "loss of power equivalent to that of discarding one-third to two-thirds of the sample" (p. 253). It also obscures nonlinear relationships, and although it reduces statistical power, it can also increase the risks of false positives (type I errors) when two or more continuous variables are dichotomized and used as predictors in regression analyses (Austin & Brunner, 2004; Maxwell & Delaney, 1993).

The loss of power can be particularly problematic in treatment outcome studies. Imagine a study on the effect of REBT on depression compared to a control group. Imagine that an analysis of response rates results in a p value of .06. I am sure that many readers of this chapter can recall being frustrated with results like this. One can neither accept nor reject the null hypothesis. Often researchers hedge by reporting a "trend," but almost as often reviewers and editors ask for this equivocation to be removed. And if you accept the practice of reporting "trends," what do you do with a p value of .11 (other than wince)?

Note that the same problem can occur when continuous data are grouped into three or more categories (Streiner, 2002). For example, one might group participants on the basis of age ranges like 20–29, 30–39, etc. This might even be done by having the participants report the age group to which they belong, rather than simply report their age. The loss of power is not as great as when the data are dichotomized, but there is still a substantial loss of information that could affect the conclusions that are reached.

In addition to statistical problems, dichotomized outcomes are prone to misinterpretation (Altman & Royston, 2006; Kirsch & Moncrieff, 2007; MacCallum et al., 2002). For example, they exaggerate the difference between people classified as "responders" and those classified as "non-responders." This can lead to claims that analyses of response rates show that a non-trivial proportion of the population is helped by a particular treatment, but not by a placebo or other control procedure, despite only trivial differences in means. In fact, it sheds no new information, but instead produces an illusion of greater effectiveness. What tends to be ignored is that the difference between a "responder" and a "non-responder" can be as little as one point or a 1% reduction of symptoms on whatever continuous scale was dichotomized. If the scale has been dichotomized near the mode of a unimodal distribution, as is often the case in antidepressant trials for example, then most of the people who would be "responders" on drug, but "non-responders" on placebo, would in fact be experiencing a very small treatment benefit.

For these reasons, continuous scores of naturally continuous variables should be used as predictors and primary outcomes in both clinical trials and meta-analyses. Continuous scores, rather than categorized variables, should be used as the basis for decision making about efficacy. Dichotomization of continuous scores should be avoided, as should statistics derived from artificially dichotomized variables (e.g., odds ratios and number needed to treat). These statistics are appropriate for naturally dichotomous variables, but not for continuous variables.

Report and analyze within-group changes as well as between-group differences

Typically, meta-analyses report between-group effect sizes, but do not analyze within-group differences. While between-group differences are important and most often the appropriate primary outcome to examine, analyses of changes within each arm of the trial can supply important additional information. The importance of examining both is best understood in relation to what Harald Walach (2001) termed "the efficacy paradox," and this paradox is most easily seen in meta-analyses comparing the effectiveness of different types of treatment.

Here I will illustrate the efficacy paradox with data on the treatment of depression with antidepressants and the treatment of migraine with acupuncture. Meta-analyses of antidepressants versus placebo for the treatment of major depressive disorder (MDD) indicate standardized mean differences (SMD) ranging from 0.23 to 0.34 (Kirsch, 2019). In contrast, a Cochrane meta-analysis (Smith, Hay, & MacPherson, 2010) showed an effect size of 0.03 for acupuncture versus placebo in the treatment of MDD. Thus, it seems clear that antidepressants are more effective than acupuncture. But wait! The Cochrane meta-analysis also reported a direct comparison of selective serotonin reuptake inhibitors (SSRIs) in the treatment of MDD showed an effect size of 0.02. That shows that the acupuncture and SSRIs have virtually identical effects. How can that be? It seems like a paradox.

The paradox is only apparent. The reason for it is the difference in the effectiveness of the placebo. Different placebos have different effects. For example, the response to placebo acupuncture is greater than the response to placebo pills in the prevention of migraine (Meissner et al., 2013). This then leads to the efficacy paradox illustrated in Figure 6.1. The response to real acupuncture is greater than the response to pills containing real medication, but the treatment effect (real minus sham treatment) of pills is greater than that of acupuncture.

Report exact means and SDs for baseline, posttreatment, and difference scores

One of the most useful innovations in clinical research has been the use of meta-analyses to summarize the results of different studies addressing the same question. However, a methodological difficulty that is often faced by

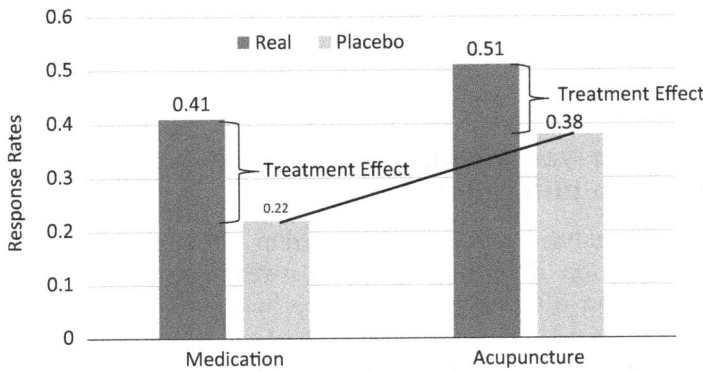

Figure 6.1 **The efficacy paradox explained**
Source: © Irving Kirsch, based on data in Meissner et al. (2013)

meta-analytic researchers is the absence of sufficient data for accurately calculating effect sizes. This problem could easily be overcome by requiring clinical trial articles to publish sample sizes and standard deviations (or standard errors and n's per group) of baseline means, posttreatment means, and change scores. Figures can be useful to provide readers with a rapid impression of the pattern of results, but actual means and standard deviations (SD) should also be reported in the text or tables. One reason for not doing this has been saving precious journal space, but with online publishing this is no longer the problem it used to be. Figures can be used in the article proper, while the exact data the figures are portraying can be published in an online supplementary file. For editors and reviewers, providing access to these data should be a requirement for publication.

Clinical trial data should include baseline scores, posttreatment scores, and change scores. It might seem that posttreatment and change scores are redundant, because either can easily be calculated from the other if baseline scores are reported. However, while this is true of means, it is not true of the SDs that are needed for calculating effect sizes. SDs of change scores are needed for the calculation of the effect sizes of between-group differences in improvement, whereas pre- and post-SDs are needed to calculate the effect sizes of within-group changes.

I must confess to having violated the precept of providing exact data for change scores as well as baseline and posttest scores (Kirsch et al., 2014). My colleagues and I reported the exact pre- and post-test data for the study, but not the change scores. I have since supplied these data to a colleague who is doing a meta-analysis and will try to be more careful in the future.

Don't control for the placebo effect in psychotherapy

The use of placebo control groups has become normative in evaluating medications and is often discussed in relation to psychotherapy research (Rosenthal & Frank, 1956). However, there are both conceptual and practical problems with the recommendation of using "placebo psychotherapy" controls (Kirsch, 1978, 2005; Kirsch, Wampold, & Kelley, 2016).

The practical problems relate to the fact that, as discussed in the previous section, all placebos are not created equal. This is tacitly recognized by the methodological practice of having placebo pills be the same size, color, taste, and perceptually identical to the active drug in all other ways. In fact, the color of the pill has been found to influence outcomes (de Craen, Roos, de Vries, & Kleijnen, 1996). This is generally possible in clinical trials of medications and most other physical interventions, but impossible in psychotherapy trials. If a "psychotherapy placebo" looks, sounds, and feels the same as the real therapy, then it is that therapy.

The solution used in many studies of behavioral and cognitive-behavioral psychotherapies has been the inclusion of "attention placebos." I will illustrate the problem with this solution with reference to an excellent study by Trexler and Karst (1972) comparing rational emotive therapy with "attention placebo" in the treatment of public speaking anxiety. The placebo in that study consisted mainly of the typical training in relaxation employed in systematic desensitization studies, but without presentation of stimulus hierarchies. Besides being a component of a well-established behavioral treatment for anxiety, relaxation training is also a recognized treatment for anxiety in and of itself (Manzoni, Pagnini, Castelnuovo, & Molinari, 2008). This does not lessen the importance of this or similar studies, but it does render them comparative treatment studies rather than studies comparing a psychological treatment to a placebo. For example, two-arm clinical trials comparing two different medications (e.g., an SSRI to a tricyclic antidepressant) without placebo controls are useful and very common (Rutherford, Sneed, & Roose, 2009), but they are not termed "placebo-controlled" trials.

The conceptual problem with "placebo-controlled" psychotherapy trials relates to the reason for using placebo controls in clinical trials. In medical research, the reason for the placebo arm is to control for the influence of psychological factors, so that the effect of the chemical constituent (or other physical characteristics in the case of interventions like surgery or acupuncture) can be evaluated. But we know in advance that the effect of a psychotherapy is, by definition, due to its psychologically active components. That is why we refer to it as a "psycho"therapy. So, what would the placebo control for? Placebos work in large part by changing expectations, but expectancy is a legitimate psychological variable. As an active treatment component, it is no less legitimate as a psychological mechanism than classical conditioning, instrumental learning, reciprocal inhibition, or challenging irrational beliefs. It is a belief concerning the future, and challenging beliefs and expectations is central to REBT and other cognitive therapies. There is, therefore, no reason to control for them when evaluating the efficacy of these treatments.

On the other hand, evaluating the role of expectations, the therapeutic relationship, and other components of the placebo effect in physical medicine is very important in psychotherapy research. But studies of this sort do not evaluate efficacy. Rather, they are mechanism studies. They address the issue of establishing which psychological processes are responsible for the efficacy of particular psychotherapies. The best way to assess the efficacy of a psychotherapy is by comparing it to a no-treatment control group or by adding it to standard treatment as usual, which is kept the same in both arms of the study. Studying expectancies, the therapeutic relationship, and similar factors that are often mislabeled as "nonspecific" can be done without reference to the placebo effect.

References

Altman, D.G., & Royston, P. (2006). The cost of dichotomising continuous variables. *BMJ, 332*(7549), 1080. doi:10.1136/bmj.332.7549.1080

Austin, P.C., & Brunner, L.J. (2004). Inflation of the type I error rate when a continuous confounding variable is categorized in logistic regression analyses. *Statistics in Medicine, 23*(7), 1159–1178. doi:10.1002/sim.1687

Cohen, J. (1983). The cost of dichotomization. *Applied Psychological Measurement, 7*(3), 249–253. doi:10.1177/014662168300700301

de Craen, A.J.M., Roos, P.J., de Vries, A.L., & Kleijnen, J. (1996). Effect of colour of drugs: Systematic review of perceived effect of drugs and their effectiveness. *British Medical Journal, 313*, 1624–1626.

Kirsch, I. (1978). The placebo effect and the cognitive-behavioral revolution. *Cognitive Therapy and Research, 2*(3), 255–264.

Kirsch, I. (2005). Placebo psychotherapy: Synonym or oxymoron? *Journal of Clinical Psychology, 61*(7), 791–803.

Kirsch, I. (2019). Placebo effect in the treatment of depression and anxiety. *Frontiers in Psychiatry, 10*(407). doi:10.3389/fpsyt.2019.00407

Kirsch, I., Kong, J., Sadler, P., Spaeth, R., Cook, A., Kaptchuk, T.J., & Gollub, R. (2014). Expectancy and conditioning in placebo analgesia: Separate or connected processes? *Psychology of Consciousness: Theory, Research, and Practice, 1*(1), 51–59. doi:10.1037/cns0000007

Kirsch, I., & Moncrieff, J. (2007). Clinical trials and the response rate illusion. *Contemporary Clinical Trials, 28*(4), 348–351.

Kirsch, I., Wampold, B.E., & Kelley, J.M. (2016). Controlling for the placebo effect in psychotherapy: Noble quest or tilting at windmills? *Psychology of Consciousness: Theory, Research, and Practice, 3*(2), 121–131. doi:10.1037/cns0000065

MacCallum, R.C., Zhang, S., Preacher, K.J., & Rucker, D.D. (2002). On the practice of dichotomization of quantitative variables. *Psychological Methods, 7*(1), 19–40. doi:10.1037/1082-989x.7.1.19

Manzoni, G.M., Pagnini, F., Castelnuovo, G., & Molinari, E. (2008). Relaxation training for anxiety: A ten-years systematic review with meta-analysis. *BMC Psychiatry, 8*(1), 41. doi:10.1186/1471-244X-8-41

Maxwell, S.E., & Delaney, H.D. (1993). Bivariate median splits and spurious statistical significance. *Psychological Bulletin, 113*(1), 181.

Meissner, K., Fässler, M., Rücker, G., Kleijnen, J., Hróbjartsson, A., Schneider, A.... Linde, K. (2013). Differential effectiveness of placebo treatments: A systematic review of migraine prophylaxis. *JAMA Internal Medicine, 173*(21), 1941–1951.

Rosenthal, D., & Frank, J.D. (1956). Psychotherapy and the placebo effect. *Psychological Bulletin, 53*(4), 294.

Royston, P., Altman, D.G., & Sauerbrei, W. (2006). Dichotomizing continuous predictors in multiple regression: A bad idea. *Statistics in Medicine, 25*(1), 127–141.

Rutherford, B.R., Sneed, J.R., & Roose, S.P. (2009). Does study design influence outcome? *Psychotherapy and Psychosomatics, 78*(3), 172–181. doi:10.1159/000209348

Smith, C.A., Hay, P.P., & MacPherson, H. (2010). Acupuncture for depression. *The Cochrane Library*. doi:10.1002/14651858.CD004046

Streiner, D.L. (2002). Breaking up is hard to do: The heartbreak of dichotomizing continuous data. *Canadian Journal of Psychiatry, 47*, 262–266.

Trexler, L.D., & Karst, T.O. (1972). Rational-emotive therapy, placebo, and no-treatment effects on public-speaking anxiety. *Journal of Abnormal Psychology, 79*(1), 60–67. doi:10.1037/h0032336

Walach, H. (2001). The efficacy paradox in randomized controlled trials of CAM and elsewhere: Beware of the placebo trap. *Journal of Alternative & Complementary Medicine, 7*(3), 213–218.

Part III

The contributions of REBT to coaching, the science of happiness, and as a philosophy of life

Chapter 7

Rational Emotive Behavioural Coaching

Present and future

Oana Alexandra David and Windy Dryden

Coaching is currently an expanding occupational domain and at the same time a field in great need of evidence-based procedures and tools. REBT is the cognitive-behavioural approach with the best fit with coaching which has been extended into Rational Emotive Behavioural Coaching (REBC), a form of cognitive-behavioural coaching (CBC). This chapter will first discuss the features of REBC and then present its types and models. The current state of the field will be then reviewed in terms of REBC and related applications and programs. The comparative efficacy of various models of REB coaching is described next. Finally, the state of the art of knowledge in terms of the evidence-based status of CBC is discussed, together with future directions of the field.

Introduction

Rational Emotive Behaviour Therapy (REBT) recognizes that a client[1] may seek help for a range of issues. For example, a client may be unhealthily angry about being treated with disrespect by their boss and also have a sense that they are not fulfilling themself at work. In working with them, the REB therapist helps them to see that, in effect, they have three problems that need attention. First, they are disturbed about their boss's behaviour towards them and, according to REBT, this *disturbance* is based on one or more rigid and extreme attitudes towards this adversity. Second, even if they were not disturbed about this adversity, they would be dissatisfied about it since it is a negative situation and they would prefer to change that situation. Third, their lack of fulfilment at work would indicate that they have an opportunity to develop themself in this area of their life. This latter issue, therefore, would fall under the heading of *development.*

REBT argues that, in this case, there is a preferred order of intervention. Thus, the REB therapist would suggest to the client that they first tackle their disturbance, then their dissatisfaction, and finally their development. Their reasoning would be as follows. When a client is disturbed about an

DOI: 10.4324/9781003081593-10

adversity, they are not in the best frame of mind to deal with that adversity or to be able to focus on their self-development. Once they have dealt with their disturbance about the adversity, the person will still be dissatisfied about it. However, this dissatisfied state will motivate them to address the adversity constructively by changing it if it can be changed or by accepting it gracefully if it can't be changed. Having done this, then the client will be able to focus on self-development (Dryden, 2021)

Traditionally, dealing with disturbance is the province of the therapist, promoting development is the province of the coach and addressing dissatisfaction may be done by either. However, today's coach needs to be trained to deal with all three areas. You may be wondering why a coach needs to be able to deal with coachee disturbance. There are two reasons for this. First, in helping the coachee deal with their development-based objective, the coachee may experience an emotionally based obstacle which they need to address to resume the pursuit of this objective. Second, a coachee with a disturbance-based problem may seek help from a coach because, in their mind, coaching is a more acceptable form of assistance to them than therapy or counselling. We will discuss both scenarios later in the chapter.

Three types of Rational Emotive Behavioural (REB) Coaching

Following on from the above, we might say that there are three types of REB coaching (Dryden, 2018a): i) development-focused REBC (DF-REBC), ii) practical problem-focused REBC (PPF-REBC), and iii) emotional problem-focused REBC (EPF-REBC). We will briefly outline each here. In doing so, we will focus on the distinctive aspects of each type of REBC. In practice, however, the REB coach will likely be called upon to move among all three types of coaching. Thus, they need to be trained and develop competence in the practice of each.

Development-focused REBC (DF-REBC)

A coachee is a good candidate for development-focused REBC when:

- The person is not in a psychologically disturbed state of mind.
- The person is not in a dissatisfied state of mind about the presence of an adversity and is not facing a practical problem.
- The person has a sense that they could develop themself in one or more areas of their life and wants to do that.

As Dryden (2018b) has outlined, DF-REBC is based on several features, most of which are in common with other approaches to coaching. Thus, the REB coach in DF-REBC helps the coachee to focus on the future, although how far in the future will depend on what the person wants to gain from coaching. In doing so, the coachee will likely state objectives that are quite general in nature. While validating such targets, the coach will strive to help the client to be as specific as possible about them later in the process. What is distinctive about DF-REBC is that several rational principles of living underpin much of it. These have been discussed by Bernard (2018a). Examples of such principles are self-direction, risk-taking and experimentation, self-acceptance and high frustration tolerance. Coaches can implement these principles in DF-REBC in two ways. First, the coach can give the coachee the full list of eleven principles and ask them to nominate those that they would like to put into practice more often in their life. Second, the coachee can choose one or more rational principles that can help them in the pursuit of their development-based coaching objectives.

As well as making use of these rational principles of living in DF-REBC, the REB coach employs several strategies that are used quite widely in cognitive-behavioural coaching (see Dryden, 2018c). These strategies help the coachee to:

- Identify and make use of their values in DF-REBC.
- Identify and use their inner strengths and resilience factors in DF-REBC.
- Develop a list of external resources that can be used when necessary during DF-REBC.
- Set meaningful development-based objectives. Here the focus is on helping the coachee to focus on one objective at a time (known as the nominated objective).
- Design and implement an action plan of relevant tasks intended to achieve the nominated objective identify and problem-solve any potential obstacles to the execution of the above tasks. Such an obstacle may be practical and/or emotional, and depending on its source the REB coach will use relevant skills from practical problem-focused REBC (PPF-REBC) or emotional problem-focused REBC (EPF-REBC) to be described below.
- Maintain progress once the coachee has achieved their nominated development-based objective.
- Pursue other development-based objectives and generalize learning.

Emotional problem-focused REBC (EPF-REBC)

As noted above, when a coachee is working towards their development-based objectives, they may encounter an obstacle, the source of which is an emotional problem. For example, if a coachee is working towards improving their entrepreneurial skills, they might experience anxiety about giving a public presentation designed to promote their business. If the person cannot work around this problem, they need to face it and deal with it effectively, and this is where the coach will use EPF-REBC.

Here, the coach will use the same skills as the REB therapist and do so within the context of the *ABC* framework (see Chapter 1). Thus, the coach will help the coachee to imagine giving a public presentation and to get in touch with their anxiety (C) as they do so. Doing this will enable the coach to help the coachee to identify the aspect of the public presentation situation about which they are most anxious. This represents the *A* or adversity. The coach then helps the coachee to understand the *B–C* connection, where *B* stands for the rigid/extreme basic attitudes that mediate between *A* and *C*. Once the coachee has understood this connection, the coach can help them to identify and examine the specific rigid/extreme attitudes that account for their anxiety and change these to their flexible/non-extreme attitude alternatives. The coach then helps the coachee to revisit giving a public presentation in their imagination, while encouraging them to rehearse their flexible/non-extreme attitudes as they focus on the adversity that featured in their problem. The coach suggests that the coachee does such mental rehearsal until they can try out the solution in real life.

Once the REB coach has helped the coachee to deal with this obstacle, the two of them can return to DF-REBC, and the coachee can resume the pursuit of their development-based objective of improving their entrepreneurial skills. If they experience further emotionally based obstacles, the two can return temporarily to EPF-REBC.

So far, we have discussed the situation where the main focus of the coaching work is developmental (i.e. DF-REBC) and where the coaching dyad makes use of EPF-REBC whenever an emotionally based obstacle arises which requires their collective attention. However, as mentioned earlier, it also happens that a person may seek coaching for their emotional problems because, for that individual, coaching is an acceptable form of help where counselling and psychotherapy are not. The question arises here, 'Should the coach accept the person for coaching under these circumstances?' One view is that the coach should not do so. This view is based on the idea that coaching and psychotherapy are discrete forms of help. As coaching is a development-based activity, the coach should not deal with a coachee's emotional problems, particularly if this is the exclusive focus for the work.

Perhaps because Rational Emotive Behavioural Coaching (REBC) emerged from Rational Emotive Behaviour Therapy (REBT) and it is likely that the REB coach is also a trained therapist, then the answer to the question as to whether the coach should see the person for coaching is yes if the coach has the relevant training and the requisite skills to do so.

Cavanagh (2005) outlined several guidelines to help coaches decide whether to offer coaching help to a coachee who has an emotional problem that may help the REB coach in this respect. Cavanagh would suggest that the REB coach should help a person with an emotional problem:

- When the emotional problem is of recent origin or if it occurs intermittently.
- When the coachee's emotional, behavioural, and/or thinking responses to the relevant adversity lie within a mild to moderate range of disturbance.
- When the coachee's emotional problem is limited to a particular situation or aspect of the person's life.

Cavanagh (2005) also noted that the coachee might meet the above three criteria with respect to the emotional problem for which they are seeking help, but still not be suitable for coaching because of their high level of defensiveness concerning the problem. Also, if the person has failed to address the problem several times before in different ways, then this may be a contraindication for coaching.

Our view is that Cavanagh's criteria are particularly useful when the coach has had some training in dealing with a coachee's emotional problem, but only in the range detailed in the above criteria. REB coaches with more extensive training in the application of REBT to more complex psychological issues would agree to see the coachee with such emotional problems when the person has sought coaching rather than psychotherapy for these problems. The concern of such coaches would be to provide help to the coachee, and as such they would not be concerned if this help was called 'coaching', 'counselling' or 'psychotherapy'. These coaches are coachee-focused and not profession-focused. Profession-focused coaching organizations keen to promote the distinctive nature of development-based coaching and to contrast this with the emotional problem-based work which is predominantly the province of counselling and psychotherapy would discourage coaches from accepting coachees in this scenario.

Practical problem-focused REBC (PPF-REBC)

We consider a practical problem to be the crystallization of an aspect of the coachee's life with which they are dissatisfied, but about which they are not (or no longer) emotionally disturbed. Here, the person would be looking to change this unsatisfactory state of affairs, if indeed it can be changed. Also, a practical problem exists where a coachee may be confused about an issue and would welcome an opportunity to discuss this with a coach. However, again, they are not emotionally disturbed about this issue.

There are three scenarios where the REB coach may be called upon to help a coachee with a practical problem:

- Where the person is seeking coaching specifically for help with that practical problem.
- Where, during DF-REBC, the person experiences an obstacle to the pursuit of their development-based objective that is practical rather than emotional.
- When the coachee has sought coaching for an emotional problem and has been helped through EPF-REBC to the point where they are no longer emotionally disturbed about the adversity that featured in their emotional issue. However, if the adversity is still present, the person may well be dissatisfied about it.

In helping the coachee to address a practical problem in what we call practical problem-focused REBT (PPF-REBC), the coach may use one of several useful frameworks (or models) to guide their work. One such framework is called the 'PRACTICE Problem-Solving Framework' (Palmer, 2008), which we outline in Table 7.1.

Using the PRACTICE framework

In using the PRACTICE framework, the coach begins by helping the coachee to identify and specify the nature of the problem ('problem identification'). In the next stage, the coach helps the coachee to set a realistic goal concerning the practical problem ('realistic, relevant goal development'). Then, the coach helps the coachee to brainstorm possible solutions to the problem, making sure not to duplicate previous attempts to solve the problem that were ineffective ('alternative potential solutions generated'). The coach then helps the coachee to stand back and evaluate these solutions ('consideration of potential solutions'). In doing so, the coach encourages the coachee:

- To consider the short- and long-term advantages of each potential solution.
- To think to what extent each solution is consistent with their relevant values.
- To reflect on whether or not they have the requisite skills to implement each potential solution.
- To judge to what extent they can incorporate each solution into their life.

Once the coachee has considered each potential solution, the coach encourages them to select the solution that seems the most likely to be effective and that they are most likely to implement. It is important to note here that the coachee may make a selection that is most likely to bear fruit, but they may not be able to implement it. Thus, the emphasis is on choosing a solution that is most feasible ('target most feasible potential solution').

Table 7.1 The **PRACTICE** problem-solving framework

	Thinking steps	Examples of problem-solving thinking
P	**P**roblem identification	What is the problem or issue that I need to focus on?
R	**R**ealistic, relevant goal development	What are the goals or objectives that I can realistically work towards, ones that will make a real difference for me?
A	**A**lternative potential solutions generated	– What have I tried already that has not worked? – Were there any elements of what I tried that were helpful on which I can build? – What are the possible ways that I can solve the problem or reach my goal or objective?
C	**C**onsideration of potential solutions	– What do I think of each of the potential solutions? (E.g. what are their consequences? Are they consistent with my values? What other aspects of each possible solution do I have to consider?)
T	**T**arget most feasible potential solution	Having looked at each potential solution and its consequences, which is likely to be the most feasible one that I can select?
I	**I**mplementation of chosen potential solution	How am I going to best implement the chosen potential solution?
C	**C**onsolidation of the chosen potential solution	How am I going to ensure that I have given the chosen potential solution the best chance to see if it yields the results I want?
E	**E**valuation	How successful was the potential solution? If it was, it becomes the solution. If not, I need to try another potential solution until I find one that works.

Source: Adapted from Palmer (2008).

The next step is for the coach to help the coachee to implement the chosen solution, using some kind of prior rehearsal to see how it feels to implement the solution before doing so in real life ('implementation of the chosen potential solution'). The coachee then implements the solution and may make modifications to it based on their experience of using it. Also, before judging its effectiveness, the coachee may need to give the chosen solution a fair chance to work ('consolidation of the chosen potential solution'). Finally, the coachee needs to evaluate the effectiveness of the selected solution ('evaluation'). If the problem still exists, then the coachee may decide to choose another solution or to accept, but not like, the existence of the problem. This latter approach needs to be taken if the practical problem cannot be changed, at least by the coachee.

Applications of REBC

Applications of REBC have been developed and described for many domains of life (see Bernard & David, 2018), such as personal, professional, health or parenting. Among its applications, life coaching is the closest to the original REBT model and has extended the original theory based on its positive programs, such as Rational Emotive Education and consultation (Vernon, 1994) and positive psychology theory. In life REBC, the coachee receives support in attaining life-related goals, such as higher life satisfaction or better life–work balance. For life developmental goals, the coach makes use of the eleven rational principles for living a happy life described by Bernard (2018a), while for emotional problem-focused or practical-problem focused life goals the coach will provide support on changing the irrational beliefs and implementing practical solutions, using various models (e.g., GRAPE,[2] ABC, PRACTICE, described earlier in this chapter).

Another domain of REBC application is organizational coaching, which is based on REBT developments such as Rational Effectiveness Training (RET; DiMattia, 1990) and the work of Ellis (1972) on executive leadership. RET is the first comprehensive model specifying how to apply REBC principles in the workplace. Organizational applications of REBC can be further separated into executive REBC, managerial REBC, or performance REBC.

Executive REBC (Dudău, Sălăgean, & Sava, 2018) refers to offering guidance to the top management of companies on attaining performance and change-related goals. Executive REBC has evolved on the basis of the rational model of leadership proposed by Ellis (1972). Essential leadership strengths such as rational sensitivity, concentration, discipline, rational decisions, effective communication and unconditional acceptance are mapped and cultivated. The Freeman–Gavita Prescriptive Executive Coaching model (Gavita, Freeman, & Sava, 2012) uses an integrative and multi-modal framework based on an initial multi-source assessment on which a prescriptive profile is extracted with recommendations for change. Starting from the strengths and weaknesses areas, goals are approached using REBC for developing problematic areas and capitalizing on the strengths of the executive.

Managerial REBC (David & Cimpean, 2018) refers to the use of coaching by managers as a development tool with their team members. The Rational Leadership Program is an REBC program developed by David (David & Matu, 2013; David, 2016) that includes both group training and executive coaching directed to improve leadership and build managerial coaching skills. Managers learn REBC coaching skills and practise it in this program based on shadowing sessions with their collaborators, and then receive feedback from the coach.

The REBC-based performance coaching has evolved on the basis of the high performance mindset at work (HPMW; Bernard, 2018b), integrating REBT theory with positive psychology (e.g., character strengths, psychological capital). Performance REBC uses a *high performance capability framework* and focuses on developing the *architecture of the high performance mindset*. The HPMW starts with a survey for identifying commitments, supporting beliefs and behavioural strengths of the coachee, and in a second step the coach uses the results for designing an individual action plan for the coachee. Great emphasis is put on the support of the coach in strengthening commitments of the coachee and in planning how to deal with tough situations at work.

Health REBC is a coaching application used to help clients in changing their lifestyle and in maintaining it (David, 2019). Coachees bring to health REBC goals such as losing weight, improving their fitness or implementing a nutritional plan. Parenting and family REBC makes use of parenting and family theories to support clients in attaining goals related to these fields, such as better management of child misbehaviour or couple satisfaction (David, Cardos, & Oltean, 2019).

The empirical status of REBC

While the practice of coaching has surpassed the evolution of evidence-based practices in this field, recently more research results have been published. Published meta-analyses (see Jones, Woods, & Guillaume, 2016; Theeboom, Beersma, & van Vianen, 2014) have shown that coaching brings moderate to high effect size outcomes in the workplace, strong effect sizes for individual level performance, and medium for the organizational.

It is worth mentioning from the beginning that REBC has started with a scientific advantage given by the empirical support already received by its theory with positive applications relevant to coaching, such as REE, RET and REBT for the workplace (see DiMattia, 1990; Trip, Vernon, & McMahon, 2007). David and Szamoskozi (2011) conducted a meta-analysis on CBT effectiveness in the workplace and found that REBT had the larger effect sizes. Among the outcomes, high effect sizes were documented for changes in irrationality and medium changes for emotional distress and its consequences after participating in workplace REBT. A recent meta-analysis was conducted to investigate the efficacy of cognitive-behavioural coaching (CBC), including REBC (see Lorint & David, under review). Some 26 articles were included in the analysis that investigated CBC using a within or between-subjects design and were published in peer-review journals. CBC was found to have an overall positive impact of moderate magnitude, with high level improvements on performance and low to medium improvements on abilities, affective and cognitive changes. Also, the analysis of moderators has shown that CBC is effective regardless of the method or format of delivery, or approach of CBC, which were specified as REBC, CBC or solution-focused CBC.

Effectiveness of the REBC process models

The effectiveness of various REBC and CBC models was investigated in several studies. The generic ABC(DEF) model of EPF-REBC, the main model of REBT, is widely used in therapy. The efficacy of the ABC model was investigated as a self-coaching and personal development tool for students enrolled in an REBC course (David et al., 2014). One hundred and five students used the ABC(DEF) form for monitoring and carrying out their established action plans. Results have shown that participants using the model reported at the end of the course lower levels of depressed mood and improved work performance. Changes in their irrational beliefs and the quality of their homework tasks were found as mechanisms of change for their outcomes. The specific components of the ABC(DEF) model that were related to changes in outcomes were investigated in a qualitative study, where the forms were coded by external raters (David & Cobeanu, 2015). Pragmatic cognitive restructuring was most frequently used by trainees and the most effective in helping change dysfunctional emotions into functional ones. These results offer support for the positive effects of using the ABC(DEF) model in REBC.

In another recent study, Comsa and David (under review) investigated the comparative efficacy of the GROW (solution focused and widely used) versus PRACTICE (problem solving and REBT-based) models in coaching. In the coaching literature, it was claimed that a solution-focused approach would be more suitable for coaching and the problem solving approach only for therapy. Our results supported the efficacy of both models without obtaining major differences in terms of their outcomes. Thus, the superiority of the solution focused model was not supported by our empirical investigation.

Based on the research conducted on REBC so far, one can conclude that REBC has strong support for effectiveness and is making use of evidence-based theory, models and programmes.

Future directions of REBC

REBC research

Although REBC has good empirical support, conclusions regarding its effectiveness need to be tempered since there are important limitations to the published research in terms of the studies design. Indeed, most studies conducted to date have used within-subjects design and many studies are underpowered. Thus, REBC and coaching research in general need to overcome these limitations and make use of sound methodologies, and investigate the mechanisms of change. Future studies need to use designs and adequate measures that allow clear conclusions in terms of both REBC efficacy and effectiveness. This is not an easy task, however, given the characteristics of both coaching settings and the clients (high status participants, organizational contracts, private funding). Moreover, the REBC and CBC fields need to develop their own methodologies (e.g. multi-rater measures) since, as suggested by Stober and Grant (2006), it might be that methods specific to the clinical field might not be the most adequate.

Technology-based REBC

Given the wide usage of technologies by coachees, various types of technologies have been used to deliver coaching/CBC from its beginnings, including online coaching, telephone coaching and email coaching. Moreover, REBC and CBC are suited for being offered through online guided or unguided applications, given their structured, directive and active approaches and their already implemented and tested protocols in the therapeutic field.

Most of the available tools focus on coaching emotion regulation skills, rational thinking, problem solving, relaxation or positive emotions. We describe below a few innovative tools that are based on REBC and have been preliminarily documented as effective, such as the PsyPills app, the REThink online serious game and the roboRETMAN device.

PsyPills app is a smartphone-based standalone tool for coaching stress resilience.[3] Using the self-reported stress rating entered by the user, the app provides a prescription with rational statements in the form of 'psychological pills' that aim to reduce acute emotional distress. The statements are derived from REBT theory and are included in a psychological prescription. The app is conceptualized as an automated 'personal coach' to be used for immediate stress relief. It was recently tested and found effective in reducing distress in a pilot study investigating its usage during the first six months (David & David, 2019).

REThink is an online serious game based on REBC strategies which was developed to promote psychological resilience among children and adolescents by coaching emotion regulation skills based on game tasks (e.g., rational thinking skills and relaxation skills).[4] REThink is meant to be used primarily as a standalone application where the superhero of Rationalia planet, the RETMAN character, is the user's guide and acts as a facilitator of the emotional skills and rational thinking.[5] The game action is divided into seven levels, each level having a different goal for skills development and saving the Earth from the powers of Irrationalius: emotional recognition, connection between beliefs and emotions, changing irrational beliefs, emotional control, problem solving, relaxation, and well-being. The game was tested in a randomized clinical trial and found to be effective in improving emotion-regulation skills in youth (David, Cardos, & Matu, 2019a,b) and will be extended for use by adults in various settings.

The RoboRETMAN is a robotic device that has been developed on the basis of REBT/C to coach specific emotional skills in young children aged 4 to10. The device is built on the action figure of the same superhero RETMAN character and offers rational statements by reading them verbally (e.g. 'It is bad but not catastrophic to feel this way') to children in distress (e.g. feeling anxiety). The child selects and shows a radiofrequency card depicting their emotion to the robotic device and a rational statement is played for this specific emotion. The functionalities of the roboRETMAN are currently being tested and updated, and experimental studies are ongoing.

Although technology-based CBC services and tools are increasingly available, the empirical research concerning their efficacy and effectiveness is still in its infancy. There are a number of studies that report promising results for the technology-based REBC presented above but more research is needed to document the results and mechanisms.

Practice and training in REBC

Among the major difficulties of the coaching field are the folk psychology practices that are still prevalent and the lack of consensus on important characteristics of coaching (e.g., approaches, directivity, training level). These difficulties reflect also in the practice and theory of REBC and CBC, making it difficult to define it and to be taken seriously by the scientific community. More specific difficulties are related to its specialized language and sophisticated theory, which make it difficult to disseminate it to the coaching practitioners/professionals outside the psychology and psychotherapy fields and to render it attractive outside academia.

REBC has a number of strengths which have the potential to support its development and flourishing, including: theory, techniques and models that are evidence-based and its high suitability for the needs of clients, existing technology-based tools and validated measures. The future of REBC needs, however, to transcend the current stage of divergences and move to deeper understanding and collaboration. This applies to its definition, characteristics, practice standards (e.g., training needed) and credentialing. The International Association of Cognitive Behavioral Coaching (IACBC)[6] is the first international body, established in 2009, with the mission to contribute through its activities to the development of the field. The first congress of CBC was organized in 2014 in Cluj-Napoca and gathered together the board of the IACBC and a workforce of experts and practitioners interested in developing the field (David, 2014, 2016). One of the main focuses of the IACBC for the following years is to make REBC and CBC understood as an evidence-based approach (i.e., reducing the stigma for the CBT practitioners who associate it with the folk practices of coaching) and contribute to the progress of knowledge in the field by supporting high quality research, training and credentialing for CBC practitioners. Another important focus is emphasizing collaboration with the main stakeholders in the more general coaching field, such as coaching academic groups and already established organizations.

Finding common ground is not an easy task in a world that favours more the business of coaching, competition for market requests and rapid certification. However, the future of REBC lies in finding means for collaboration, with the common goal of supporting the growth of the field, reflected in high quality research and the regulated practice of REBC, which will allow the promotion of REBC as an evidence-based coaching approach.

Notes

1 In this chapter, we will refer to a 'client' when that person is consulting a Rational Emotive Behaviour Therapist and to a 'coachee' when that person is consulting a Rational Emotive Behavioural Coach.
2 GRAPE stands for 'Goals, Reflection, Action Planning, Evaluation' (see Bernard, 2018b).
3 See https://itunes.apple.com/us/app/psypills/id589004229?mt=8.
4 See http://rethink.info.ro/index.html for details.
5 See www.retman.ro.
6 See www.iacbc.org.

References

Bernard, M.E. (2018a). Rationality in coaching. In M.E. Bernard & O.A. David (Eds.), *Coaching for living: Theory, techniques and applications* (pp. 51–66). New York: Springer.

Bernard, M.E. (2018b). Coaching high workplace performance. In M.E. Bernard & O.A. David (Eds.), *Coaching for living: Theory, techniques and applications* (pp. 295–324). New York: Springer.

Bernard, M.E., & David, O.A. (Eds.) (2018). *Coaching for living: Theory, techniques and applications*. New York: Springer.

Cavanagh, M.J. (2005). Mental-health issues and challenging clients in executive coaching. In M.J. Cavanagh, A.M. Grant, & T. Kemp (Eds.), *Evidence-based coaching: Theory, research and practice from the behavioural sciences* (pp. 21–36). Bowen Hills, QLD: Australian Academic Press.

Comsa, L., & David, O.A. (under review). GROW or PRACTICE in coaching? That is the question. Manuscript under review.

David, A.R., & Szamoskozi, S. (2011). A meta-analytical study on the effects of cognitive behavioral techniques for reducing distress in organizations. *Journal of Cognitive and Behavioral Psychotherapies,11*(2), 221–236.

David, O.A. (Ed.). (2014). *Congress book of the 1st International Congress of Cognitive Behavioral Coaching*. Cluj-Napoca: Presa Universitară Clujeană.

David, O.A. (2016). The foundations and evolution of cognitive behavioral coaching in organizations: An interview with Dominic DiMattia. *Journal of Rational-Emotive and Cognitive-Behavioral Therapy, 34*(4), 282–288.

David, O.A. (2019). REBT in coaching: Theory, practice, research, measurement, prevention and promotion. In M. Bernard and W. Dryden (Eds.), *Advances in REBT: Theory, practice, research, measurement, prevention and promotion*. New York: Springer.

David, O.A., Cardos, R.A.I., & Matu, S.A. (2019a). Is REThink therapeutic game effective in preventing emotional disorders in children and adolescents? Outcomes of a randomized clinical trial. *European Child and Adolescent Psychiatry*. doi: 10.1007/s00787-018-1192-2

David, O.A., Cardos, R.A.I., & Matu, S.A. (2019b). Changes in irrational beliefs are responsible for the efficacy of the REThink therapeutic game in preventing emotional disorders in children and adolescents: Mechanisms of change analysis of a randomized clinical trial. *European Child and Adolescent Psychiatry*. doi: 10.1007/s00787-018-1195-z

David, O.A., Cardos, R.A.I., & Oltean, H.-R. (2019). REBT and parenting intervention. In M. Bernard & W. Dryden (Eds.), *Advances in REBT: Theory, practice, research, measurement, prevention and promotion*. New York: Springer.

David, O.A., & Cimpean, A. (2018). Managerial coaching and rational leadership. In M.E. Bernard & O.A. David (Eds.), *Coaching for rational living: Theory, techniques and applications* (pp. 325–341). New York: Springer (ISBN 978-3-319-74067-6).

David, O.A., & Cobeanu, O. (2015). Evidence-based training in cognitive-behavioural coaching: Can personal development bring less distress and better performance? *British Journal of Guidance &Counselling, 44*, 12–25.

David, O.A., & David, D. (2019). Managing distress using mobile prescriptions of psychological pills: A first 6-month effectiveness study of the PsyPills app. *Frontiers in Psychiatry, 10*, 201.

David, O.A., Ionicioiu, I., Imbarus, C.A., & Sava, F.A. (2016). Coaching banking managers through the financial crisis: Effects on stress, resilience, and performance. *Journal of Rational-Emotive and Cognitive-Behavioral Therapy, 34*(4), 267–281.

David, O.A., & Matu, S.A. (2013). How to tell if managers are good coaches and how to help them improve during adversity? The Managerial Coaching Assessment System and the Rational Managerial Coaching Program. *Journal of Cognitive and Behavioral Psychotherapies, 13*, 259–274.

David, O.A., Matu, A., Pintea, S., Cotet, C., & Nagy, D. (2014). Cognitive-behavioral processes based on using the ABC analysis by trainees for their personal development. *Journal of Rational-Emotive and Cognitive-Behavioral Therapy, 32*(3), 198–215.

DiMattia, D. (1990). *Rational effectiveness training: Increasing productivity at work*. New York: Institute for Rational Emotive Therapy.

Dryden, W. (2018a). A step-based framework for practice. In M.E. Bernard & O.A. David (Eds.), *Coaching for rational living: Theory, techniques, applications* (pp. 143–179). New York: Springer.

Dryden, W. (2018b). Life coaching. In M.E. Bernard & O.A. David (Eds.), *Coaching for rational living: Theory, techniques, applications* (pp. 213–228). New York: Springer.

Dryden, W. (2018c). *Cognitive-emotive-behavioural coaching: A flexible and pluralistic approach.* Abingdon, Oxon: Routledge.

Dryden, W. (2021). *Rational emotive behaviour therapy: Distinctive Features. Third edition.* Abingdon, Oxon: Routledge.

Dudău, D.P., Sălăgean, N., Sava, F.A. (2018). Executive coaching. In M.E. Bernard & O. David (Eds.), *Coaching for living: Theory, techniques and applications* (pp. 343–360). New York: Springer.

Ellis A. (1972). *Executive leadership: A rational approach.* New York: Institute for Rational Living.

Gavita, O.A., Freeman, A., & Sava, A.F. (2012). The development and validation of the Freeman–Gavita Prescriptive Executive Coaching (PEC) Multi-Rater Assessment. *Journal of Cognitive and Behavioral Psychotherapies, 12*(2), 159–174.

Jones, R.J., Woods, S.A., & Guillaume, Y.R. (2016). The effectiveness of workplace coaching: A meta-analysis of learning and performance outcomes from coaching. *Journal of Occupational and Organizational Psychology, 89,* 249–277.

Lorint, C. & David, O.A. (under review). Is cognitive-behavioral coaching an empirically supported approach to coaching? A meta-analysis to investigate its outcomes and moderators.

Palmer, S. (2008). The PRACTICE model of coaching: Towards a solution-focused approach. *Coaching Psychology International, 1*(1), 4–6.

Stober, D.R. & Grant, A.M. (Eds.). (2006). *Evidence based coaching handbook: Putting best practices to work for your clients.* Hoboken, NJ: John Wiley & Sons Inc.

Theeboom, T., Beersma, B., & van Vianen, A.E. (2014). Does coaching work? A meta-analysis on the effects of coaching on individual level outcomes in an organizational context. *Journal of Positive Psychology, 9*(1), 1–18.

Trip, S., Vernon, A., & McMahon, J. (2007). Effectiveness of rational-emotive education: A quantitative meta-analytical study. *Journal of Cognitive & Behavioral Psychotherapies, 7*(1), 81–93.

Vernon, A. (1994). Rational-emotive consultation: A model for implementing rational-emotive education. In M.E. Bernard & R. DiGiuseppe (Eds.), *Rational-emotive consultation in applied settings: School psychology.* Hillsdale, NJ: Lawrence Erlbaum Associates.

Chapter 8

Rational Emotive Behavior Therapy and happiness

Aurora Szentágotai-Tătar, Andrei C. Miu, Diana-Mirela Nechita, and Daniel David

Although Rational Emotive Behavior Therapy (REBT) is best known as a theory and treatment of emotional problems, it has always had a distinct interest in happiness and in how it can be achieved. The current chapter reviews the REBT perspective on well-being by focusing on two major issues: what goals people should choose in order to be happy, and how these goals should be formulated and pursued. We argue that, by its emphasis on reducing irrational thinking and by teaching a rational outlook on life and its challenges, REBT promotes profound, long-lasting well-being. By encouraging both short-term pleasure and long-term fulfillment, it also promotes well-rounded, balanced well-being. The unique contribution of REBT and the evidence supporting it are analyzed in light of recent findings regarding well-being.

Traditionally focused on reducing symptoms and deficits, cognitive behavioral psychotherapies (CBT) are increasingly orienting toward developing strengths and resilience and fostering positive emotions (e.g., Ingram & Snyder, 2006). However, the oldest form of CBT, Rational Emotive Behavior Therapy (REBT), founded by Albert Ellis in the 1950s, has always had a distinct interest not only in helping people overcome their problems, but also in teaching and encouraging them to pursue self-development and happiness (Ellis, 1984; Ellis & Becker, 1982; Ellis & Dryden, 1997). This chapter describes the REBT perspective on well-being and on how it can be achieved, putting it in the context of recent findings on happiness and fulfillment. Following the lead of prominent authors in the field (e.g. Diener et al., 2018), we use the concepts of happiness and well-being interchangeably throughout the chapter.

Emotional health first

REBT sees people as complex, biosocial organisms with a strong tendency to establish and pursue a wide range of goals and purposes (Dryden, David, & Ellis, 2010). As there is no universal road to well-being, goals should be

DOI: 10.4324/9781003081593-11

established in accordance with individual preferences and talents, keeping in mind that, in the long run, happiness is most likely to be related to goals that reduce emotional pain, maximize comfort and pleasure, and lead to healthy relationships and to excellence at work and in other activities (Bernard, 2011; Ellis, 1991). While the question of *what* goals people should pursue has been central to discussions on well-being both in philosophy and in psychology, unique to REBT is the idea that *how* goals are formulated is just as important, if not more important, than the content of goals (Szentágotai-Tătar, Cândea, & David, 2019; Szentágotai-Tătar & David, 2013).

REBT maintains that cognitions play a key role in generating emotions and behaviors, and distinguishes between two types of biologically based thinking patterns: *rational* and *irrational* (Ellis, 1991; Ellis, 1995; Ellis & Dryden, 1997). The core of irrationality is the rigid formulation of goals and desires, expressed in the dogmatic insistence that certain conditions must or must not exist. These demands lead to three other irrational beliefs: awfulizing (i.e., extreme, dichotomous evaluations of negative events as worse than they absolutely should be), low frustration tolerance (i.e., beliefs that one cannot tolerate or bear an event or set of circumstances) and global evaluations of self, others and life (i.e., the tendency to rate a specific trait, action or situation according to a standard of desirability or worth, and then apply this evaluation to the person or life as a whole) (MacInnes, 2004).

Irrational thinking is an important obstacle to well-being by generating problematic emotions and behaviors and by sabotaging the person's goals (DiGiuseppe & Doyle, 2019). Indeed, a meta-analysis of 83 studies found a positive association between irrational beliefs and general distress, and irrational beliefs and negative emotions such as anxiety, depression, anger and guilt (Vîslă et al., 2016). Moreover, a study that involved over 450 participants showed that global evaluation of the self and demanding approval and perfection were negative predictors of joviality, self-assurance and life satisfaction (Ciarocchi, 2004). Thus, attaining mental health, by vigorously and persistently fighting the self-defeating tendency of irrational thinking, is a key condition of well-being, which is otherwise undermined by problematic negative emotions and maladaptive behaviors (Dryden, 2009; Ellis, 1995; Ellis, 2001).

At the heart of mental health lie flexible, non-dogmatic formulations of personal goals and desires (Dryden et al., 2010). These are assertions of what the person wants, coupled with acceptance of the fact that we cannot insist that we absolutely get what we want. The rational derivatives of preferences are non-awfulizing (i.e., concluding that circumstances may be "bad" but not "awful" when preferences are not met, which allows for the fact that worse outcomes are possible and relies on a continuum of badness rather than a dichotomous judgment), high frustration tolerance (i.e., beliefs that events may be difficult to tolerate, but they are not intolerable), and unconditional acceptance of self, others, and life (i.e., beliefs that although people do bad things and circumstances may be bad, they cannot be globally rated as bad, which leads to the acceptance of self and others as fallible human beings, and to the acceptance of life conditions as they are) (Dryden, 2002; Dryden et al., 2010).

While more research on the relation between rational thinking and positive outcomes is needed, existing data support the REBT proposal that rationality promotes happiness by helping people reach their goals or formulate new ones when old ones cannot be attained (Dryden et al., 2010). A recent study on 397 participants found rationality to explain 33% of self-reported happiness levels and 40% of self-reported optimism (Oltean et al., 2018). Among rational beliefs, self-acceptance was a significant predictor of both happiness and optimism, while preferences were indirect predictors, through self-acceptance (Oltean et al., 2018). Two other studies reported positive associations between unconditional self-acceptance, happiness and life satisfaction (Chamberlain & Haaga, 2001), and unconditional self-acceptance and psychological well-being (MacInnes, 2006). On the other hand, Davies (2006) found that unconditional self-acceptance was significantly negatively related with neuroticism, one of the most important negative predictors of well-being (Steel, Schmidt, & Shultz, 2008).

Achieving emotional health is, thus, an essential first step toward well-being, but it does not entirely overlap with well-being (Ellis & Blau, 1998). According to REBT, people can be free from suffering, but still far from happy. Therefore, after learning how to be less disturbed, they should focus on discovering what they enjoy in life and try to get more of that, and what they dislike in life and try to have less of that (Ellis & Blau, 1998).

Short-term satisfaction and long-term fulfillment

Answers to the question of what happiness is tend to cluster around two related but distinct perspectives, stemming from different philosophies: the hedonic view and the eudaimonic view (Keyes, Shmotkin, & Ryff, 2002; Ryan & Deci, 2001; Waterman, 1993). The hedonic view equates happiness with pleasure, enjoyment and satisfaction, resulting from fulfilling one's desires and valued outcomes in a variety of realms, and with comfort, painlessness and ease (Huta, 2017b; Huta & Ryan, 2010). The mindsets typically associated with hedonic experiences are a focus on the self, on the present moment, on the tangible, and on getting and consuming what one desires (Huta, 2017b). Positive affect, satisfaction and low negative affect are among the most commonly used indexes of well-being from this perspective (Huta, 2017b; Kesebir & Diener, 2008; Ryan & Deci, 2001).

The eudaimonic view rejects the idea of reducing well-being to enjoyment, seeing it rather as a life of purpose, of cultivating personal strengths, of living in accordance with individual potentialities, which ultimately lead to flourishing and fulfillment (Ryff & Singer, 2006; Waterman, 1993). While definitions of eudaimonia vary more widely than those of hedonia, according to an analysis by Huta and Waterman (2014) four contents appear to feature in most of them: meaning/value/relevance to a broader context, personal growth/self-realization, excellence/ethics/quality, and authenticity/autonomy/integration. Mindsets typically associated with eudaimonia are a balance between self-focus and a focus on others, between a focus on the present and a focus on the future, and a tendency to be guided by abstract concepts and to concentrate on cultivating what the person values (Huta, 2017b).

Most psychological accounts of well-being view hedonia and eudaimonia as complementary and consider that both are needed in order for people to flourish (Huta, 2015, 2017b). REBT is no exception, as it describes two types of well-being, both legitimately pursued: short-term satisfaction and long-term fulfillment (Bernard, 2011; Ellis & Harper, 1975). Short-term satisfaction is defined in terms of feelings of pleasure, which can be achieved through involvement in a wide range of activities (Bernard, 2011; Ellis & Becker, 1982). While significant pleasure can be sometimes derived from passive involvement (e.g., watching TV), the active involvement in creative and absorbing activities is a much more likely and efficient source (Ellis & Becker, 1982).

Long-term fulfillment is also conceptualized as positive emotions, resulting from the realization of individual potential, striving toward excellence and self-actualization (Bernard, 2011; Ellis, 1995). According to REBT, all humans are born with constructive and creative tendencies and with the ability to increase their self-fulfilling tendencies (Ellis, 1973). However, self-actualization involves a choice, an active and effortful quest, and it is intimately related to goals (Ellis & Blau, 1998; Ellis & Dryden, 1997). One of the main goals that leads to it is to seek for spontaneous ways of living, which helps people discover enjoyable things that can become future goals. To become self-actualized, people should constantly ask themselves what they really like and dislike, how they can experiment and discover what they prefer or do not prefer, what future effects their preferences have, and what are the best ways to achieve their preferences and avoid their dislikes (Ellis & Blau, 1998). As they are free from demands and cognitive rigidity, self-actualizing people are open to alternative paths to happiness and self-realization (Ellis & Blau, 1998). Inspired by Abrahm Maslow, Carl Rogers and Alfred Korzybski, Ellis describes the self-actualizing person as having the following characteristics: nonconformity and individuality; self-awareness; acceptance of ambiguity and uncertainty; tolerance; acceptance of human animality; commitment and intrinsic enjoyment; creativity and originality; social interest and ethical trust; enlightened self-interest; self-direction; flexibility and scientific outlook; unconditional self-acceptance;

risk-taking and experimenting; long-range hedonism; work and practice (Ellis & Blau 1998).

Although the importance of hedonic and eudaimonic motives for well-being is an ongoing discussion in the literature (Huta & Ryan, 2010; Huta, 2017a), research that has looked at how they relate to happiness confirms the REBT perspective that they are both significant contributors to the good life. People who pursue both hedonia and eudaimonia report higher levels of well-being and higher levels of mental health than people who pursue only one (Huta & Ryan, 2010; Keyes, 2002; Peterson, Park, & Seligman, 2005). Moreover, hedonia and eudaimonia fill different niches of well-being (Huta, 2017b), and therefore people who pursue both are at an advantage. Thus, hedonic motives are more related to positive affect, carefreeness and low negative affect, while eudaimonic motives are more related to meaning, self-connectedness and elevating experiences (Huta & Ryan, 2010). The pursuit of hedonia is mainly related to individual well-being (Huta & Ryan, 2010; Peterson et al., 2005), while the pursuit of eudaimonia is linked both with personal well-being and with the tendency to care for the well-being of others and the surrounding world (Huta, 2012; Pearce, Huta, & Voloaca, 2020). Finally, there is some evidence suggesting that hedonia is more related to short-term happiness, while eudaimonia is more related to long-term happiness (Huta & Ryan, 2010; Pearce et al., 2020).

REBT note on positive and negative emotions

Positive affect is a key element in definitions of well-being (Diener et al., 1999; Diener, Oishi, & Tay, 2018), and factor analyses indicate that it accounts for a large proportion of the variance in the hedonic factor (Huta, 2017b). REBT recognizes the importance of positive emotions and encourages people to discover and constantly experiment with things that can bring them joy (Ellis & Becker, 1982; Ellis & Dryden, 1997). However, REBT is unique in proposing that positive emotions can be *functional* or *dysfunctional,* depending on the beliefs they result from (Dryden et al., 2010). Positive emotions that stem from irrational thinking (e.g., elation after being praised, resulting from the belief that "people must absolutely appreciate my work, and I will not take it otherwise") are seen as dysfunctional, as they reinforce the underlying irrational beliefs and focus people on short-term rather than long-term benefits (David et al., 2005). Positive emotions that result from rational beliefs (joy after being praised, related to the belief that "I would like people to appreciate my work, and this time they did, but I accept that it might not always happen") are seen as helpful or functional and essential to well-being (Ellis & Blau, 1998).

Research in REBT has mainly focused on negative emotions, and the distinction between functional and dysfunctional positive emotions is almost unexplored. We believe that their understanding would not only influence the way we conceptualize well-being, but also clarify the role of positive emotions in psychological disorders (Szentágotai-Tătar et al., 2019). For example, pride plays a critical role in several domains of psychological functioning, particularly in prosocial behavior and achievement-related behavior (Tracy & Robins, 2007). However, pride can be also profoundly dysfunctional, and associated with aggression, interpersonal problems and a variety of self-destructive behaviors, as in the case of narcissism (Tracy & Robins, 2004). It has already been proposed that the difference between healthy and unhealthy (i.e., hubristic) pride lies in the appraisals each involves (Tracy & Robins, 2004). Therefore, focusing on rational/irrational beliefs as antecedents could definitely contribute to a better understanding of the adaptive and maladaptive facets of this emotion, as well as of other positive emotions.

In discussing well-being and self-actualization, Ellis warns against the dangers of demanding that we absolutely must attain them, and against the negative effects of blaming ourselves or others when we do not (Ellis & Blau, 1998). An interesting line of research, unrelated to REBT, supports these ideas. For example, data show that people who value happiness to an extreme degree, endorsing affirmations such as "How happy I am at any given moment says a lot about how worthwhile my life is," "If I don't feel happy, maybe there is something wrong with me," and "To have a meaningful life, I need to be happy all the time" (Mauss et al., 2011), report lower well-being and more loneliness (Mauss et al., 2011; Mauss et al., 2012). Moreover, the extreme valuation of happiness has been proposed as a general risk factor for mood disturbance (Ford, Mauss, & Grueber, 2015), as it is associated with depressive symptoms and a diagnosis of depression both in adults and in adolescents (Ford et al., 2014), and with more severe symptoms, increased risk and worse prognosis of bipolar disorder (Ford et al., 2015; Gentzler et al., 2019).

Alongside positive emotions, low negative affect is another element that usually features in definitions of well-being (Diener et al., 2018; Huta, 2017b). Research suggests that the two are independent factors and should be addressed separately (Diener et al., 1999), and that negative affect has closer links with hedonia than with eudaimonia (Huta, 2013). Across cultures, the experience of positive emotions is related to happiness judgments more strongly than the absence of negative emotions, which indicates that positive experience is an important route to greater happiness and life satisfaction (Kuppens, Realo, & Diener, 2008). However, it is also clear that, under certain conditions, having negative emotions is more reflective of healthy functioning than not having them or avoiding them (Ryan & Deci, 2001; Shallcross et al., 2010).

As in the case of positive emotions, REBT maintains that not all negative emotions are created equal, and distinguishes between functional negative emotions, resulting from rational beliefs regarding negative situations, and dysfunctional negative emotions, generated by irrational beliefs following negative life events. Although in the same family, as they are the product of qualitatively different ways of thinking, functional and dysfunctional negative emotions are considered qualitatively, not just quantitatively, different (David, 2003; Ellis & DiGiuseppe, 1993). While dysfunctional negative emotions are associated with psychological disturbance and are incompatible with happiness (see Vîslă et al., 2016 for a meta-analysis), functional negative emotions are reflective of good mental health under conditions of adversity. They elicit efficient problem solving, adaptive coping and social interactions (DiGiuseppe & Doyle, 2019) and are compatible with well-being (Bernard et al., 2010). Existing data confirm quantitative (e.g., Cramer & Fong, 1991) and qualitative (e.g., David, Schnur, & Birk, 2004) differences between functional and dysfunctional negative emotions, but the role of functional negative emotions in well-being has yet to be determined. However, a recent meta-analysis on the relation between rational beliefs and psychological distress found a moderate negative association between the two (Oltean & David, 2018). The authors conclude that their results confirm the protective function of rational beliefs against emotional disturbance, as hypothesized by REBT (Oltean & David, 2018).

REBT recommendations for a happy life

REBT outlines several principles that should guide people in their pursuit of happiness and self-actualization. These principles are discussed in detail elsewhere (see Bernard et al., 2010; DiGiuseppe & Doyle, 2019; Ellis & Becker, 1982; Ellis & Bernard, 1985; Ellis & Dryden, 1997), but we revisit some of them in light of recent research on well-being.

Self-interest and social interest

Two basic rules of morality should guide people's behavior, according to REBT. The first one is "be true or kind to yourself" (Ellis & Becker, 1982). In terms of seeking happiness, this translates into putting personal well-being first, before the well-being of others (Ellis & Becker, 1982; Ellis & Bernard, 1985). The choice of making ourselves as happy as we can is closely linked to the choice to stay alive, because it is unlikely for people to want to be alive if they experience constant misery. People who discount this first rule are likely to end up in emotional trouble because they expect others to reciprocate their sacrifice, which usually does not happen, because they can be exploited by others, or because their self-sacrificing behavior results from the irrational demand of being loved and approved (Ellis & Becker, 1982). On the other hand, people who put their needs slightly before those of others are more likely to lead an authentic and honest existence, more likely to make a valuable contribution toward changing the world for the better, and ultimately more likely to make people around them happy (Ellis & Becker, 1982).

Research confirms that people are most satisfied with their lives, experience most positive emotions and least negative emotions when their needs are fulfilled (e.g., Tay & Diener, 2011). Furthermore, progress toward and attainment of personal goals predict increased well-being, which persists in time and sustains future goal attainment (Sheldon & Elliot, 1999; Sheldon & Hauser-Marko, 2001). This effect is dependent on goal type (i.e., intrinsic vs. extrinsic motives) and reasons for pursuing the goal (i.e., autonomous vs. controlled motives). While intrinsic and autonomous motives are positively related to well-being, extrinsic and controlled motives are significant negative predictors of well-being (Sheldon et al., 2004). Finally, findings also support the idea that happy individuals make the ones around them happy. For example, longitudinal data from the Framingham Heart Study indicate that people's happiness extends up to three degrees of separation (for example, to friends of one's friends), and that people who are surrounded by many happy people are more likely to become happy in the future than those who are not (Fowler & Christakis, 2008).

The second rule that people should abide by in order to be happy is "do not harm others" (Ellis & Becker, 1982). Self-interest should be fused with social interest, and a balance found between putting one's own needs first and a sincere preoccupation for the needs of others, whose well-being should be put a close second to our own (Ellis & Becker, 1982). In Ellis's words: "strive for personal happiness in a social world. Individual and social living inextricably merge, so that the summit of your individuality and freedom involves real concern for others. Be yourself while helping others." (Ellis & Becker, 1982, p. 165). The benefits of focusing on others' well-being is well documented in the literature, and research shows that altruistic behavior is associated with significant and lasting benefits in terms of emotional and physical health (e.g., Brown et al., 2003; Brown, Consedine, & Magai, 2005; Schwartz et al., 2003). It is beyond the scope of this chapter to review this evidence. We only mention that a recent study that included participants from 166 nations found that the world's happiest people (i.e. those who score 9 or 10 on a 0–10-point scale) virtually all report having strong social relationships and high quality social lives (Diener et al., 2018).

Self-direction, frustration tolerance and effort toward realistic goals

Self-direction involves people assuming responsibility for their own happiness, rather than placing it on others or relying on others for it (Bernard et al., 2010; Ellis & Dryden, 1997). A distinction is made in REBT between having the will and having the willpower to pursue happiness (Ellis, 1999). Having the will refers to making the choice, expressing the decision of working toward being happy; having the willpower is harder, and it involves persisting in trying to reach a goal, taking the appropriate actions and doing them again and again, until the goal is reached (Ellis, 1999). This requires frustration tolerance, that is, preferring, but not demanding, that life provides you with what you want easily, and understanding that, in order to achieve pleasant results in the long term, you sometimes have to tolerate discomfort in the short run (Bernard et al., 2010).While low frustration tolerance discourages people from contending with unpleasant circumstances, and short-circuits their ability to confront obstacles to goal attainment, high frustration tolerance promotes active efforts to confront or eliminate obstacles to happiness and achievement (Dryden, 2002).

The role of having the will is supported by the literature showing that intentional activity is one of the most efficient ways of increasing well-being (Sheldon & Lyubomirsky, 2019), and that happiness boosting activities are most beneficial for people who explicitly express a desire to become happier (Lyubomirsky et al., 2011). Where willpower is concerned, long-term benefits of these activities have mainly been found in individuals who invest energy into reaching their goals, and then continuous and sustained effort into maintaining gains (Sheldon et al., 2010). Grit, defined as perseverance and passion for long-term goals, which entails working strenuously toward challenges and maintaining effort and interest over time despite failures or adversities (Duckworth et al., 2007), is related not only to achievement, but also to well-being, both hedonic and eudaimonic (Disabato, Goodman, & Kashdan, 2019; Jiang et al., 2019; Vainio & Daukantaité, 2016).

While REBT strongly encourages people to assume responsibility for their happiness, and to invest time and effort into getting the things they want, it also warns against the dangers of striving for the unattainable (Ellis & Dryden, 1997). Accepting that we will probably not get everything we desire and going for realistic, attainable goals is also a prerequisite of well-being (Ellis & Dryden, 1997). Indeed, data confirm that the persistent pursuit of need-satisfying goals leads to happiness when there is a way of reaching them (Sheldon et al., 2010), but that it becomes maladaptive in the case of unattainable goals (Miller & Wrosch, 2007).

Flexibility and scientific thinking

Healthy individuals are flexible in their thinking, open to change, and pluralistic in their views of others (Ellis & Dryden, 1997). When people adopt a flexible perspective, they will not become disturbed, even if confronted with unpleasant conditions or negative life events (Dryden et al., 2010). Psychological inflexibility (i.e., the tendency to hold on to rigid, dogmatic beliefs in the form of demands) is the central element of emotional and behavioral disturbance (Dryden et al., 2010). According to REBT, there are three main types of demands that create problems for people: (1) demands that they should perform well, (2) demands that others must treat them nicely, and (3) demands that living conditions must be free of hassles and that life should be fair (Ellis, 2003).

The relation between psychological inflexibility and dysfunctional emotions and behaviors is well-established (e.g., David, Schnur, & Belloiu, 2002; David et al., 2005; Szentágotai-Tătar & Jones, 2010). Inflexibility is also a negative predictor of well-being (e.g., Ciarrochi, 2004). On the other, hand, recent evidence shows that flexible, preferential thinking is positively related to happiness (Oltean et al., 2018)

REBT advocates scientific thinking as one of the most efficient antidotes against the psychological misery resulting from inflexibility (Ellis, 1995). Scientific thinking involves testing of our beliefs against evidence from reality and replacing them with valid ideas, should they prove wrong (Ellis, 1995). This approach not only prevents emotional problems by precluding the escalation of preferences into demands, but is also the way to eliminate emotional problems in people who, for various reasons, have endorsed dogmatic demands. Scientific thinking entails passing our beliefs through the following filters: establishing if they are realistic or factual; establishing if they are logical; determining if they are flexible and non-rigid; establishing if they can be falsified; determining if they prove deservingness; and evaluating if they will lead to good and happy outcomes for ourselves and for others (Ellis, 1995).

Acceptance

REBT was the first form of cognitive behavioral therapy to emphasize the crucial role of acceptance for emotional health and well-being. Ellis argues that conditional acceptance, that is, only accepting ourselves, others or life under certain conditions, is "one of the greatest sicknesses" (Ellis, 1999, p. 50), responsible for most human disturbance (Ellis, 2005), and that unconditional acceptance is one of the most important lessons REBT teaches (Ellis, 1999). Three major forms of acceptance are described in REBT: (1) fully accepting ourselves, whether or not we succeed at important tasks, and whether or not we are approved by others (i.e., unconditional self-acceptance); (2) fully accepting others, whether or not they act fairly or competently (i.e., unconditional other acceptance); and (3) fully accepting life, whether or not it is fortunate or unfortunate (i.e., unconditional life acceptance) (Ellis, 2005).

Unconditional self- and other acceptance are based on the assumption that a person cannot be given a single global rating that defines her and her worth. They involve acknowledging that we are complex beings, subject to constant change, that defy rating, while at the same time accepting that we are essentially fallible (Dryden & Neenan, 2004; Ellis & Dryden, 1997). However, unconditional acceptance allows people to rate their and others' actions and traits, and encourages such ratings as a means of personal change and improvement (Ellis, 1999). Ultimately, it helps people become free and concentrate on enjoying their lives, rather than on proving how good or how bad they or others are (Ellis, 1999).

Studies confirm the positive relation between self-acceptance, life satisfaction, happiness (Chamberlain & Haaga, 2001), psychological well-being (MacInnes, 2006) and optimism (Oltean et al., 2018), and self-acceptance's negative relation with neuroticism, anxiety and depression (Davies, 2006). Conversely, global self-rating has a negative effect on most components of well-being and is associated with dysfunctional negative emotions (e.g., DiGiuseppe & Tafrate, 2007), relationship and marital problems (Addis & Bernard, 2002; Möller & De Beer, 1998; Möller, Rabe, & Nortje, 2001) and poor goal setting and pursuit (Flett et al., 2003). Although, to our knowledge, unconditional other acceptance has not been studied in relation to well-being, blaming others has been linked to stress, anxiety, depression (Martin & Dahlen, 2005) and aggression (Stuewig et al., 2010).

Accepting that we live in a world of probabilities, where absolute certainties are unlikely to ever exist, is, according to REBT, another condition for well-being (Ellis & Dryden, 1997). REBT therefore recommends that we learn to see uncertainty as a challenge, not as a threat, and learn to live with it if we want to reach important goals and enjoy life as much as possible (Ellis, 1999; Ellis & Dryden, 1997). A recent meta-analysis found that irrational beliefs related to certainty are significant predictors of dysfunctional automatic thoughts (Şoflău & David, 2017). Intolerance of uncertainty has been linked to a variety of other problems that significantly affect well-being, such as pathological worry (Koerner & Dugas, 2008), symptoms of phobia, depression, panic and obsessive-compulsive disorder (Gentes & Meron Ruscio, 2011; McEvoy & Mahoney, 2012), and reduced well-being in the context of life changes (Bardi, Guerra, & Ramdeny, 2009).

Commitment to absorbing activities and risk taking

Getting vitally absorbed into something is, according to REBT, synonymous with happiness and contentment (Ellis & Harper, 1975). This requires, in the first place, overcoming the inertia resulting from irrational beliefs related to failure, effort and responsibility for well-being (Ellis & Harper, 1975). It then involves experimenting with a wide range of activities that fall into three main types of pursuits: (1) loving or feeling absorbed in other people, (2) creating or getting absorbed in things and (3) philosophizing or being absorbed by ideas (Ellis & Harper, 1975). In the ideal situation, people invest and become absorbed both in other people and in things, as each comes with its own advantages. However, if at certain times one is not within reach, significant pleasure and meaning can be derived from getting wholeheartedly involved in the other (Ellis & Harper, 1975). Research confirms that intentional activity is one of the most efficient ways of enduringly influencing happiness levels (Lyubomirsky, Sheldon, & Schkade, 2005). Involvement often leads to flow (Csikszentmihalyi, 1990), which is related not only with hedonic and eudaimonic well-being (Bassi et al., 2013), but also with efficient coping with stressful situations (Rankin, Walsh, & Sweeny, 2018). A recent study has identified that high-flow and high-well-being inducing activities center around the following five themes: romantic relationships, spirituality, creative activities, physical activity and engagement with others (Isham, Gatersleben, & Jackson, 2018).

REBT also encourages risk taking and experimenting with activities that entail a high likelihood of failure (Ellis & Harper, 1975). This helps fight fear of failure and performance anxiety and, at the same time, can lead to the discovery of new sources of well-being (Bernard et al., 2010). Indeed, there is evidence showing that people who plan their daily goals so as to avoid their worst fears report significantly lower levels of happiness than those who plan so as to reach broader life objectives (King, Richards, & Stemmerich, 1998). Also, studies looking at the relations between personality traits and happiness indicate that openness to experience is a robust predictor of self-actualization (Keyes et al., 2002).

Conclusions

Although REBT is best known as a theory and treatment of emotional problems, it also has a distinct interest in happiness and in how it can be achieved (Ellis, 1999). By its focus on reducing irrational thinking and teaching a rational outlook on life and its challenges, REBT promotes profound, long-lasting well-being. It also teaches a balanced and well-rounded perspective on happiness by emphasizing both pleasure and self-actualization. While studies have mainly focused on assessing the efficacy of REBT in reducing emotional disturbance, data also support its potential for increasing well-being. For example, a recent meta-analysis found a significant beneficial effect of REBT on quality of life, in a variety of clinical and non-clinical populations (David et al., 2017). Moreover, REBT school interventions are associated with increases in well-being, social-emotional competences and academic achievement in children and adolescents (Ashdown & Bernard, 2012; Bernard & Walton, 2011; Shannon & Allen, 1998).

In order to better exploit REBT insights into the nature of happiness, and to strengthen its position as a valuable tool for increasing well-being, important topics for future research include: further exploring the relation between rational/irrational thinking and indicators of well-being; describing the nature and correlates of functional and dysfunctional positive emotions; evaluating the impact of interventions based on REBT principles on increasing happiness; and establishing the efficacy of REBT in preventing psychopathology.

References

Addis, J., & Bernard, M.E. (2002). Marital adjustment and irrational beliefs. *Journal of Rational-Emotive & Cognitive-Behavior Therapy, 2*(1), 3–13.

Ashdown, D.M., & Bernard, M.E. (2012). Can explicit instruction in social and emotional learning skills benefit the social-emotional development, well-being and academic achievement of young children? *Early Childhood Education Journal, 39*(6), 397–405.

Bardi, A., Guerra, V.M., & Ramdeny, G.S.D. (2009). Openness and ambiguity intolerance: Their differential relations to well-being in the context of academic life transition. *Personality and Individual Differences, 47*(3), 219–223.

Bassi, M., Steca, P., Monzani, D., Greco, A., & Delle Fave, A. (2013). Personality and optimal experience in adolescence: Implications for well-being and development. *Journal of Happiness Studies, 15*(4), 829–842.

Bernard, M.E. (2011). *Rationality and the pursuit of happiness: The legacy of Albert Ellis*. Chichester: Wiley-Blackwell.

Bernard, M.E., Froh, J.J., DiGiuseppe, R., Joyce, M.R., & Dryden, W. (2010). Albert Ellis: Unsung hero of positive psychology. *Journal of Positive Psychology, 5*(4), 302–310.

Bernard, M.E. & Walton, K. (2011). The effect of You Can Do It! Education in six schools on student perceptions of wellbeing, teaching, learning, and relationships. *Journal of Student Wellbeing, 5*(1), 22–37.

Brown, S.L., Nesse, R.M., Vinokur, A.D., & Smith, D.M. (2003). Providing social support may be more beneficial than receiving it: Results from a prospective study of mortality. *Psychological Science, 14*(4), 320–327.

Brown, W.M., Consedine, N.S., & Magai, C. (2005). Altruism relates to health in an ethnically diverse sample of older adults. *Journals of Gerontology Series B: Psychological Sciences and Social Sciences, 60*(3), 143–152.

Chamberlain, J.M., & Haaga, D.A.F. (2001). Unconditional self-acceptance and psychological health. *Journal of Rational-Emotive and Cognitive-Behavior Therapy, 19*(3), 163–176.

Ciarrochi, J. (2004). Relationship between dysfunctional beliefs and positive and negative indices of well-being: A critical evaluation of the common beliefs survey-III. *Journal of Rational-Emotive & Cognitive-Behavior Therapy, 22*(3), 171–188.

Cramer, D., & Fong, J. (1991). Effects of rational and irrational beliefs on intensity and "inappropriateness" of feelings: A test of rational-emotive theory. *Cognitive Therapy and Research, 15*(4), 319–329.

Csikszentmihalyi, M. (1990). *Flow: The psychology of optimal experience.* New York: Harper Collins.

David, D. (2003). Rational emotive behavior therapy (REBT): The view of a cognitive psychologist. In W. Dryden (Ed.), *Rational emotive behaviour therapy: Theoretical developments* (pp. 130–159). London: Brunner-Routledge.

David, D., Coteţ, C., Matu, S., Mogoaşe, C., & Ştefan, S. (2017). 50 years of rational-emotive and cognitive-behavioral therapy: A systematic review and meta-analysis. *Journal of Clinical Psychology, 74*(3), 304–318.

David, D., Schnur, J., & Belloiu, A. (2002). Another search for "hot" cognitions: Appraisal, irrational beliefs, attributions, and their relation to emotion. *Journal of Rational Emotive & Cognitive Behavior Therapy, 20*(2), 93–131.

David, D., Schnur, J., & Birk, J. (2004). Functional and dysfunctional feelings in Ellis' cognitive theory of emotion: An empirical analysis. *Cognition and Emotion, 18*(6), 869–880.

David, D., Szentágotai, A., Kállay, E., & Macavei, B. (2005). A synopsis of Rational-Emotive Behavior Therapy (REBT): Fundamental and applied research. *Journal of Rational-Emotive & Cognitive-Behavior Therapy, 23*(3), 175–221.

Davies, M.F. (2006). Irrational beliefs and unconditional self-acceptance. I. Correlational evidence linking the key features of REBT. *Journal of Rational-Emotive & Cognitive-Behavior Therapy, 24*(2), 113–124.

Diener, E., Oishi, S., & Tay, L. (2018). Advances in subjective well-being research. *Nature Human Behaviour, 2*(4), 253–260.

Diener, E., Seligman, M.P.E., Choi, H., & Oishi, S. (2018). Happiest people revisited. *Perspective on Psychological Science, 13*(2), 176–184.

Diener, E., Suh, E.M., Lucas, R.E., & Smith, H.L. (1999). Subjective well-being: Three decades of progress. *Psychological Bulletin, 125*(2), 276–302.

DiGiuseppe, R.A., & Doyle, K.A. (2019). Rational emotive behavior therapy. In K.S. Dobson & D.J.A. Dozois (Eds.), *Handbook of cognitive-behavioral therapies* (4th ed., pp. 191–207). New York: Guilford Press.

DiGiuseppe, R.A., & Tafrate, R.C. (2007). *Understanding anger disorder.* New York: Oxford University Press.

Disabato, D.J., Goodman, F.R., & Kashdan, T.B. (2019). Is grit relevant to well-being and strengths? Evidence across the globe for separating perseverance of effort and consistency of interests. *Journal of Personality, 87*(2), 194–211.

Dryden, W. (2002). *Fundamentals of rational emotive behaviour therapy.* London: Whurr Publishers Ltd.

Dryden, W. (2009). *Understanding emotional problems: The REBT perspective.* East Sussex: Routledge.

Dryden, W., David, D., & Ellis, A. (2010). Rational emotive behavior therapy. In K.S. Dobson (Ed.), *Handbook of cognitive-behavioral therapies* (3rd ed., pp. 226–276). New York: Guilford Press.

Dryden, W., & Neenan, M. (2004). *The rational emotive behavioural approach to therapeutic change.* London: Sage Publications Ltd.

Duckworth, A.L., Peterson, C., Matthews, M.D., & Kelly, D.R. (2007). Grit: Perseverance and passion for long-term goals. *Journal of Personality and Social Psychology, 92*(6), 1087–1101.

Ellis, A. (1973). *Humanistic psychotherapy.* New York: McGraw Hill.

Ellis, A. (1984). The essence of RET. *Journal of Rational-Emotive Therapy, 2*(1), 19–25.

Ellis, A. (1991). The revised ABCs or rational-emotive therapy (RET). *Journal of Rational-Emotive and Cognitive-Behavior Therapy, 9*(3), 139–172.

Ellis, A. (1995). *How to stubbornly refuse to make yourself miserable about anything – yes, anything.* Secaucus, NJ: Lyle Stuart.

Ellis, A. (1999). *How to make yourself happy and remarkably less disturbable.* Atascadero, CA: Impact Publishers.

Ellis, A. (2001). *Overcoming destructive beliefs, feelings and behaviors: New directions for rational emotive behavior therapy.* New York: Prometheus.

Ellis, A. (2003). Differentiating preferential from exaggerated and musturbatory beliefs in rational emotive behavior therapy. In W. Dryden (Ed.), *Rational emotive behaviour therapy: Theoretical developments* (pp. 22–34). New York: Brunner Routledge.

Ellis, A. (2005). Can rational-emotive behavior therapy (REBT) and acceptance and commitment therapy (ACT) resolve their differences and be integrated? *Journal of Rational-Emotive & Cognitive-Behavior Therapy, 23*(2), 153–168.

Ellis, A., & Becker, I. (1982). *A guide to personal happiness.* North Hollywood, CA: Wilshire Books.

Ellis, A., & Bernard, M.E. (1985). What is rational-emotive therapy (RET)? In A. Ellis & M.E. Bernard (Eds.), *Clinical applications of rational-emotive therapy* (pp. 1–30). New York: Plenum Press.

Ellis, A., & Blau, S. (Eds.) (1998). *The Albert Ellis reader: A guide to well-being using rational emotive behavior therapy.* Secaucus, NJ: Citadel Press.

Ellis, A., & DiGiuseppe, R.A. (1993). Are inappropriate or dysfunctional feelings in rational-emotive therapy qualitative or quantitative? *Cognitive Therapy & Research, 17*(5), 471–477.

Ellis, A. & Dryden, W. (1997). *The practice of Rational Emotive Behavior Therapy* (2nd ed.). New York: Springer Publishing Company.

Ellis, A., & Harper, R.A. (1975). *A new guide to rational living.* North Hollywood, CA: Wilshire Books.

Flett, G.L., Besser, A., Davis, R.A., & Hewitt, P. (2003). Dimensions of perfectionism, unconditional self-acceptance, and depression. *Journal of Rational-Emotive & Cognitive-Behavior Therapy, 21*(2), 119–138.

Ford, B.Q., Mauss, I., & Gruber, J. (2015). Valuing happiness is associated with bipolar disorder. *Emotion, 15*(2), 211–222.

Ford, B.Q., Shallcross, A.J., Mauss, I.B., Floerke, V.A., & Gruber, J. (2014). Desperately seeking happiness: Valuing happiness is associated with symptoms and diagnosis of depression. *Journal of Social and Clinical Psychology, 33*(10), 890–905.

Fowler, J.H., & Christakis, N.A. (2008). Dynamic spread of happiness in a large social network: Longitudinal analysis over 20 years in the Framingham Heart Study. *British Medical Journal, 337*, a2338.

Gentes, E.L., & Meron Ruscio, A. (2011). A meta-analysis of the relation of intolerance of uncertainty to symptoms of generalized anxiety disorder, major depressive disorder, and obsessive-compulsive disorder. *Clinical Psychology Review, 31*(6), 923–933.

Gentzler, A.L., Palmer, C.A., Ford, B.Q., Moran, K.M., & Mauss, I.B. (2019). Valuing happiness in youth: Associations with depressive symptoms and well-being. *Journal of Applied Developmental Psychology, 62*(2), 220–230.

Huta, V. (2012). Linking people's pursuit of eudaimonia and hedonia with characteristics of their parents: Parenting styles, verbally endorsed values, and role modeling. *Journal of Happiness Studies, 13*(1), 47–61.

Huta, V. (2013). Pursuing eudaimonia versus hedonia: Distinctions, similarities, and relationships. In A. Waterman (Ed.), *The best within us: Positive psychology perspectives on eudaimonic functioning* (pp. 139–158).Washington, DC: APA Books.

Huta, V. (2015). The complementary roles of eudaimonia and hedonia and how they can be pursued in practice. In S. Joseph (Ed.), *Positive psychology in practice: Promoting human flourishing in work, health, education, and everyday life* (2nd ed., pp. 159–182). Hoboken, NJ: Wiley.

Huta, V. (2017a). Eudaimonia versus hedonia: What is the difference? And is it real? *International Journal of Existential Positive Psychology, 7*(2), 1–8.

Huta, V. (2017b). An overview of hedonic and eudaimonic well-being concepts. In L. Reinecke & M.B. Oliver (Eds.), *The Routledge handbook of media use and well-being: International perspectives on theory and research on positive media effects* (pp. 14–33). Abingdon: Routledge/Taylor & Francis Group.

Huta, V., & Ryan, R.M. (2010). Pursuing pleasure or virtue: The differential and overlapping well-being benefits of hedonic and eudaimonic motives. *Journal of Happiness Studies, 11*(6), 735–762.

Huta, V., & Waterman, A. (2014). Eudaimonia and its distinction from hedonia: Developing a classification and terminology for understanding conceptual and operational definitions. *Journal of Happiness Studies, 15*(6), 1425–1456.

Ingram, R.E., & Snyder, C.R (2006). Blending the good with the bad: Integrating positive psychology and cognitive psychotherapy. *Journal of Cognitive Psychotherapy: An International Quarterly, 20*(2), 117–122.

Isham, A., Gatersleben, B., & Jackson, T. (2018). Flow activities as a route of living well with less. *Environment and Behavior, 51*(4), 431–461.

Jiang, W., Jiang, J., Du, X., Gu, D., Sun, Y., & Zhang, Z. (2019). Striving and happiness: Between- and within-person-level associations among grit, need satisfaction and subjective well-being. *Journal of Positive Psychology, 15*(4), 543–555.

Kesebir, P., & Diener, E. (2008). In pursuit of happiness: Empirical answers to philosophical questions. *Perspectives on Psychological Science, 3*(2), 117–125.

Keyes, C.L.M. (2002). The mental health continuum. From languishing to flourishing in life. *Journal of Health and Social Research, 43*(2), 207–222.

Keyes, C.L.M., Shmotkin, D., & Ryff, C.D. (2002). Optimizing well-being: The empirical encounter of two traditions. *Journal of Personality and Social Psychology, 82*(6), 1007–1022.

King, L.A., Richards, J.H., & Stemmerich, E. (1998). Daily goals, life goals and worst fears: Means, ends, and subjective well-being. *Journal of Personality, 66*(5), 713–744.

Koerner, N., & Dugas, M.J. (2008). An investigation of appraisals in individuals vulnerable to excessive worry: The role of intolerance of uncertainty. *Cognitive Therapy and Research, 32*(5), 619–638.

Kuppens, P., Realo, A., & Diener, E. (2008). The role of positive and negative emotions in life satisfaction judgment across nations. *Journal of Personality and Social Psychology, 95*(1), 66–75.

Lyubomirsky, S., Dickerhoof, R., Boehm, J.K., & Sheldon, K.M. (2011). Becoming happier takes both a will and a proper way: An experimental longitudinal intervention to boost well-being. *Emotion, 11*(2), 391–402.

Lyubomirsky, S., Sheldon, K.M., & Schkade, D. (2005). Pursuing happiness: The architecture of sustainable change. *Review of General Psychology, 9*(2), 111–131.

MacInnes, D.L. (2004). The theories underpinning rational emotive behaviour therapy. *International Journal of Nursing Studies, 41*(6), 685–695.

MacInnes, D.L. (2006). Self-esteem and self-acceptance: An examination into their relationship and their effect on psychological health. *Journal of Psychiatric and Mental Health Nursing, 13*(5), 483–389.

Martin, R.C., & Dahlen, E.R. (2005). Cognitive emotion regulation in the prediction of depression, anxiety, stress, and anger. *Personality and Individual Differences, 39*(7), 1249–1260.

Mauss, I.B., Savino, N.S., Anderson, C.L., Weisbuch, M., Tamir, M., & Laudenslager, M.L. (2012). The pursuit of happiness can be lonely. *Emotion, 12*(5), 908–912.

Mauss, I.B., Tamir, M., Anderson, C.L., & Savino, N.S. (2011). Can seeking happiness make people happy? Paradoxical effects of valuing happiness. *Emotion, 11*(4), 807–815.

McEvoy, P.M., & Mahoney, A.E.J. (2012). To be sure, to be sure: Intolerance of uncertainty mediates symptoms of various anxiety disorders and depression. *Behavior Therapy, 43*(3), 533–545.

Miller, G.E., & Wrosch, C. (2007). You've gotta know when to fold 'em: Goal disengagement and systemic inflammation in adolescence. *Psychological Science, 18*(9), 773–777.

Möller, A.T., & De Beer, Z.C. (1998). Irrational beliefs and marital conflict. *Psychological Reports, 82*(1), 155–160.

Möller, A.T., Rabe, H.M., & Nortje, C. (2001). Dysfunctional beliefs and marital conflict in distressed and non-distressed married individuals. *Journal of Rational-Emotive & Cognitive-Behavior Therapy, 19*(4), 259–270.

Oltean, H.R., & David, D.O. (2018). A meta-analysis of the relationship between rational beliefs and psychological distress. *Journal of Clinical Psychology, 74,* 883–895.

Oltean, H.R., Hyland, P., Vallières, F., & David, D. (2018). Rational beliefs, happiness and optimism: An empirical assessment of REBT's model of psychological health. *International Journal of Psychology, 54*(4), 495–500.

Pearce, K., Huta, V., & Voloaca M. (2020). How eudaimonic and hedonic orientations map onto seeing beyond "me, now, and tangible." *Journal of Positive Psychology.* DOI: 10.1080/17439760.2020.1791943

Peterson, C., Park, N., & Seligman, M.P.E. (2005). Orientations to happiness and life satisfaction: The full life versus the empty life. *Journal of Happiness Studies, 6*(1). 25–41.

Rankin, K., Walsh, L.C., & Sweeny, K. (2018). A better distraction: Exploring the benefits of flow during uncertain waiting periods. *Emotion, 19*(5), 818–828.

Ryan, R.M., & Deci, E.L. (2001). On happiness and human potentials: A review of research on hedonic and eudaimonic well-being. *Annual Review of Psychology, 52,* 141–166.

Ryff, C.D., & Singer, B.H. (2006). Know thyself and become what you are: A eudaimonic approach to psychological well-being. *Journal of Happiness Studies, 9*(1), 13–39.

Schwartz, C., Meisenhelder, J.B., Ma, Y., & Reed, G. (2003). Altruistic social interest behaviors are associated with better mental health. *Psychosomatic Medicine, 65*(5), 778–785.

Shallcross, A.J., Troy, A.S., Boland, M., & Mauss, I.B. (2010). Let it be: Accepting negative emotional experiences predicts decreased negative affect and depressive symptoms. *Behaviour Research and Therapy, 48*(9), 921–929.

Shannon, H.D., & Allen, T.W. (1998). The effectiveness of a REBT training program in increasing the performance of high school students in mathematics. *Journal of Rational-Emotive and Cognitive-Behavior Therapy, 16*(3), 197–209.

Sheldon, K.M., Abad, N., Ferguson, Y., Gunz, A., Houser-Marko, L., Nichols, C.P., & Lyubomirsky, S. (2010). Persistent pursuit of need-satisfying goals leads to increased happiness: A 6-month experimental longitudinal study. *Motivation and Emotion, 34*, 39–48.

Sheldon, K.M., & Elliot, A.J. (1999). Goal striving, need satisfaction, and longitudinal well-being: The self-concordance model. *Journal of Personality and Social Psychology, 76*(3), 482–497.

Sheldon, K.M., & Houser-Marko, L. (2001). Self-concordance, goal attainment and the pursuit of happiness: Can there be an upward spiral? *Journal of Personality and Social Psychology, 80*(1), 152–165.

Sheldon, K.M., & Lyubomirsky, S. (2019). Revisiting the sustainable happiness model and pie chart: Can happiness be successfully pursued? *Journal of Positive Psychology.* https://doi.org/10.1080/17439760.2019.1689421

Sheldon, K.M., Ryan, R.M., Deci, E.L., & Kasser, T. (2004). The independent effects of goal contents and motives on well-being: It's both what you pursue and why you pursue it. *Personality and Social Psychology Bulletin, 30*(4), 475–486.

Şoflău, R., & David, D. (2017). A meta-analytical approach of the relationship between the irrationality of beliefs and the functionality of automatic thoughts. *Cognitive Therapy and Research, 41*, 178–192.

Steel, S., Schmidt, J., & Shultz, J. (2008). Refining the relationship between personality and subjective well-being. *Psychological Bulletin, 134*, 138–161.

Stuewig, J., Tangney, J.P., Heigel, C., Harty, L., & McCloskey, L. (2010). Shaming, blaming and maiming: Functional links among the moral emotions, externalization of blame and aggression. *Journal of Research in Personality, 44*(1), 91–102.

Szentágotai-Tătar, A., Cândea D.M., & David, D. (2019). REBT and Positive Psychology. In M.E. Bernard & W. Dryden (Eds.), *Advances in REBT: Theory, practice, research, measurement, prevention and promotion* (pp. 247–266). New York: Springer.

Szentágotai-Tătar, A., & David, D. (2013). Self-acceptance and happiness. In M. Bernard (Ed.), *The strength of self-acceptance* (pp. 121–137). New York: Springer.

Szentágotai-Tătar, A., & Jones, J. (2010). The behavioral consequences of irrational beliefs. In D. David, S.J. Lynn, & A. Ellis (Eds.), *Rational and irrational beliefs: Research, theory and clinical practice* (pp. 75–97). New York: Oxford University Press.

Tay, L., & Diener, E. (2011). Needs and subjective well-being around the world. *Journal of Personality and Social Psychology, 101*(2), 354–365.

Tracy, J.L., & Robins, R.W. (2004). Putting the self into self-conscious emotions: A theoretical model. *Psychological Inquiry, 15*(2), 103–125.

Tracy, J.L., & Robins, R.W. (2007). The psychological structure of pride: A tale of two facets. *Journal of Personality and Social Psychology, 92*(3), 506–525.

Vainio, M.M., & Daukantaité, D. (2016). Grit and different aspects of well-being: Direct and indirect relationships via sense of coherence and authenticity. *Journal of Happiness Studies, 17*(5), 2119–2147.

Vîslă, A., Flückiger, C., grosse Holtforth, M., & David, D. (2016). Irrational beliefs and psychological distress: A meta-analysis. *Psychotherapy and Psychosomatics, 85,* 8–15.

Waterman, A.S. (1993). Two conceptions of happiness: Contrasts of personal expressiveness (eudaimonia) and hedonic enjoyment. *Journal of Personality and Social Psychology, 64*(4), 678–691.

Chapter 9

Rational Emotive Behavior Therapy as a philosophy of life

Walter J. Matweychuk[1]

Rational Emotive Behavior Therapy, the pioneering form of cognitive behavior therapy, is more than an evidence-based psychotherapeutic system. REBT meets the criteria for a philosophy of life as it contains both metaphysics and ethics. Unlike other CBT therapies developed in academic settings, REBT specifies essential elements of emotional health and suggests how to maximize well-being and meaning in life. Those elements include enlightened self-interest, social interest, self-direction, independent thought, unconditional self-acceptance, unconditional other-acceptance, self-responsibility for own emotional disturbance, unconditional life-acceptance, calculated risk-taking, long-term hedonism, and semantic precision. The author shows how he successfully implements these elements in his life and areas where he struggles to implement REBT effectively or consistently. These areas include his struggles with awfulizing, discomfort anxiety, and people rating. The advantages and potential disadvantages of viewing REBT as a philosophy of life are identified. The chapter closes with a discussion of how practitioners who adopt it both as evidence-based psychotherapy and as a philosophy of life can minimize these potential disadvantages.

I have practiced as a Rational Emotive Behavior Therapist for over thirty years. When I embarked on my career, I wanted to learn cognitive behavior therapy because it was a sensible treatment approach. Over time, REBT has evolved into a philosophy of life I use every day. It helps me make decisions and structures my day-to-day activity. REBT's teachings impact all aspects of my life, including my politics, views on deities, religion, death and the process of dying, and how I conduct myself in my personal and professional relationships. REBT has helped me refine my beliefs and values that have roots in my upbringing, but it has also led me to leave some behind. I have remained committed to REBT not out of loyalty to Albert Ellis. I have done so because I have not found a better way to understand myself, relate to others, and live well in a challenging world. REBT for me has gone from the psychotherapy I do to the philosophy of life I embody.

DOI: 10.4324/9781003081593-12

Ellis said that the best practitioners of REBT were those who practiced it on themselves. Ellis has written quite a bit on how he used REBT to help himself cope with different personal problems throughout his life. The list of his applications of REBT includes severe parental neglect, frequent and prolonged childhood hospitalizations, chronic physical illness including headaches and diabetes as an adult. He also used REBT to cope with his significantly diminished hearing later in life. Although he was highly efficient and forthright as an adult, earlier in his life Ellis had to apply REBT to problems with procrastination, fear of rejection from women, and fear of public speaking. As a graduate student, he had to use it to cope with his first doctoral dissertation thesis's censorship and other obstacles created by feuding faculty. As the father of cognitive behavior therapy, Ellis had to use his rational philosophy to face significant criticism from the professional community threatened by his new paradigm for psychotherapy (Ellis, 2004). Finally, once the CBT paradigm became mainstream, he had to consistently tolerate professionals who borrowed and repackaged many of his ideas without giving due credit to him (Velten, 2007).

Windy Dryden also has written on how he has used REBT to address some of his personal problems, not limited to coping with prolonged unemployment, irretrievably losing an entirely written book due to a data transfer error, and adopting and adhering to a low-fat, low-cholesterol diet (Dryden, 2013). Epictetus said, "Don't explain your philosophy. Embody it." Following the lead of Epictetus, Ellis, and Dryden, I have attempted to use REBT principles to cope with personal problems, self-actualize, and maximize the pleasure and meaning I derive in life. At this point in my life, my psychotherapeutic interventions are an extension of the philosophy I implement daily.

Although Albert Ellis initially developed REBT in 1955 to be a new, efficient and effective form of psychotherapy, it has evolved significantly over the years. In my view, it is time to argue that REBT is a philosophy of life. It certainly is an empirically supported, distinct form of cognitive behavior therapy. However, REBT's philosophical roots, explicitly stated values, and its goal of profound philosophical change make it more than the most versatile and useful pioneering CBT approach available. The time has come for REBT practitioners to proclaim that REBT is not merely an evidence-based CBT psychotherapeutic approach, but also a philosophy of life.

Definition of philosophy

If one has an understanding of how the world works and how to conduct oneself with others, one has a philosophy of life (Pigliucci, Cleary, & Kaufman, 2020). Therefore, a philosophy of life has both a metaphysics and an ethics. I will discuss the metaphysics and ethics of REBT.

Metaphysics

Metaphysics is a philosophy applied to the examination of reality and to understanding it. REBT philosophy is consistent with the principles of postmodernism and relativism. REBT is against the idea that there are absolute truths about reality. It advocates that an examination of reality and conclusions about it remain flexibly held and open to revision. REBT holds that some inferences may be better than others because of the observable data, but our views and theory may reflect our biases as much as they reflect reality itself (Dryden, 2015).

From an epistemological point of view, REBT is squarely against an authoritarian epistemology. REBT theory encourages holding hypotheses consistent with facts, not faith, nor mystical and transpersonal ideas. REBT endorses knowledge derived from the use of the scientific method. Its goal is to identify empirically supported ideas about the world, oneself, and others. It is committed to the falsification of claims and updating theories, hypotheses, and beliefs. It, therefore, promotes realistic attitudes and beliefs that help us achieve personal goals. Knowledge about the world is not gained by intuition but through replicated observation which serves to eliminate adherence to dogma (Walen, DiGiuseppe, and Dryden, 1992). REBT relies on probability to navigate "reality" and encourages people to accept that certainty does not exist and that we live in a probabilistic world.

How does REBT's metaphysics translate into my philosophy? I am a probabilistic atheist and use scientific thinking to get through life. I assume it is safe to believe that this life, and nothing more, is all that I get. If there is an afterlife, REBT's ethics will probably make me a candidate for it as these ethics are consistent with Judeo-Christian values, ethical humanism, and other major organized religions. This philosophical stance does not mean I necessarily encourage others to adopt probabilistic atheism. It does mean that I encourage others to examine aspects of their beliefs about a deity, an afterlife, and adherence to religion in a flexible, nondogmatic, non-self-condemning way if there is a reason to do this. I suggest this examination to experience healthy emotions when a patient's religious beliefs lead to unhealthy negative emotions.

Ethics

Ethics pertains to how you conduct yourself in the world with others. As a practicing psychologist, most of the problems I discuss throughout the day involve people's self-defeating reactions to other people. Humans easily upset themselves about weaknesses and mistakes, as well as the people they live and work with, know, and love. REBT is a philosophy that helps us to live well with ourselves and with others. Unlike other forms of cognitive behavior therapy, REBT has a clear stance on how one preferably should think and conduct oneself to maximize well-being (Ellis, & Dryden, 2007). This stance is perhaps the best reason to consider REBT as a philosophy of life. These elements guide my day-to-day decision making and help ensure my well-being and the meaning I derive in life.

I will now discuss REBT's explicitly stated values and how they guide me in my decision making and how I have implemented them in my life.

Enlightened self-interest

REBT's philosophy sees an essential element of emotional health as being able to put oneself first, guiltlessly and shamelessly, while holding others a close second (not a distant second) when making decisions and taking action in one's interpersonal affairs. Doing so does not mean that I must put myself first all the time. It merely means I can do so when the matter is of importance to me and I do this with due ethical regard for others. REBT philosophy liberates me because I avoid taking the position: "I must not put my interests above those of another." Thinking this way, I would likely conclude: "If I do put myself first and others second, that makes me a bad person." The result of this illogical conclusion would be self-condemning guilt. REBT philosophy argues that putting myself first does not place responsibility for my life and well-being in the hands of another (Ellis & Becker, 1982). It puts that responsibility where it belongs, in my hands. If I were to place others first and myself second, I might assume they will do likewise. In a world where resources can be in short supply, this is a dubious assumption. I also would have to assume that others know what pleases me and that others are competent and motivated to ensure my well-being – another dubious assumption. REBT philosophy encourages self-responsibility for my life. I implement this philosophy with enlightened self-interest.

How does this play out in my life? My philosophy of enlightened self-interest enabled me to choose psychology as a career instead of a safer and more lucrative career. It freed me to choose the woman I have been married to for twenty-six years. If I had not been capable of putting myself first, I would have made many different choices in both of these areas to appease my well-meaning but strong-minded father. Had I not been able to put myself first, I would never have lived in New York City for twenty years. I very well could be a practicing attorney or a physician living in the suburbs with two children, married to a different woman, and regularly attending religious services on Sunday. However, I chose to follow my path, the one just described. My self-interested choices have served me well. I have enjoyed a happy marriage, living and working in cities, and my work as a practitioner and disseminator of REBT. My life has meaning thanks to my choice to train as a psychologist, which led to my having come to know Albert Ellis and his philosophy.

Social interest

REBT philosophy sees social interest as rational and self-helping because I choose to live in a community. Because I live in a social world, it is in my long-term best interest to consider others' feelings, goals, and rights while not holding myself responsible for managing other people's emotions and lives. It is in my interest to be concerned but not overly concerned for others.

How does social interest play out in my life philosophy? I strive to model personal responsibility so that others also learn how to take care of themselves and be responsible for and manage their emotional reactions. I care about society at large. I work to disseminate REBT on Saturdays through my free Zoom Conversation Hour. I want others to learn how to manage their own emotions, deal with adversity, and have some happiness despite the unfairness and misfortune that occurs to everyone. I have a website, REBTDoctor.com, where I make audio and video on this liberating philosophy available for free so others can improve their lives. I am concerned that society does not provide emotional education. I am concerned that our modern, technologically oriented society does not teach people how to accept what cannot be changed but instead we exclusively rely on technological solutions to all our problems. I am concerned that society does not empower individuals to care for and think for themselves and reinforces too much dependency on others. I think we are too quick to hold others responsible for our lives and exert subtle social pressure on how "others" need to help individuals get through life. In my view the best way to help is by teaching a man to fish rather than giving him a fish dinner. I want to teach people emotional responsibility and how to care for and rely on themselves. Dissemination of REBT philosophy allows me to give expression to my social interest and concern.

Self-direction and independent thought

REBT argues that the emotionally healthy person considers the advice of informed others but is capable of independent thinking and makes their own decisions and takes responsibility for the consequences of those decisions. I point out that REBT teaches us how to think for ourselves rather than blindly follow family, society, religion, or other figures of authority in our lives.

How do I implement this in my life? I have pointed out how I independently chose my career despite my father's strong protests. Also, my choice of spouse and living circumstances are demonstrations of my independent thinking. Furthermore, I am choosing my path and thinking independently, thanks to REBT's philosophy regarding my lack of religious practice. I have abandoned my Catholic upbringing and the idea there is a higher power that I must worship. My time is too precious to spend attending religious services, following rituals, and accepting instruction as to how I must live according to certain commandments in order to be worthy of a heavenly afterlife. My ability to think independently is reflected in my identity as an REBT psychologist. I am probably the only REBT psychologist who identifies as such in the city of Philadelphia. REBT is not a popular way of branding and practicing as a mental health practitioner. I am the only mental health practitioner affiliated with two major universities, the University of Pennsylvania and New York University, who unabashedly identifies as an REBT practitioner. I do so because in my view REBT is different and has important advantages over generic cognitive behavior therapy. Other mental health professionals are strongly inclined to label themselves cognitive behavior therapists. However, I refuse to do this because it is an imprecise label for my therapy. REBT is a distinctive form of CBT, and the use of its name highlights it is different than generic CBT. It is essential and important to me to inform the public I teach a philosophy that helps people to face reality and accept what cannot be changed. I want people to know that I encourage disciplining one's mind and assuming personal responsibility for one's emotions and behavior while letting go of conditional self-esteem in favor of unconditional self-acceptance. I model unconditionally tolerating others while seeking to influence their behavior and unconditionally accepting life while acknowledging utopias do not exist. I want to convey that I do more than help with symptom reduction. I seek to adhere to Ellis's goal of fostering profound philosophical growth. I label myself an REBT psychologist because it assists me in my mission to educate the public that REBT is different and more robust than generic cognitive behavior therapy.

Unconditional self-acceptance

How we relate to ourselves is part of ethics when defined broadly. We preferably should consider how we relate to both ourselves and to others. REBT philosophy teaches that the "self" and all "people" are unique, complex, in a state of flux, and error-prone. We are imperfect creatures with general limitations and specific fallibilities. Consequently there are no superhumans or subhumans. People are unique, with their own goals, values, strengths, and weaknesses. These elements can be validly rated, but it is invalid to sum the parts and rate the individual overall (Ellis, 1996). REBT advocates choosing unqualified self-acceptance as the antidote for our fallible nature. This stance is unique in psychotherapy in so far as REBT places the matter of unconditional self-acceptance front and center.

How does this element of the philosophy of REBT impact my life? This element frees me to take calculated risks in my profession and my personal life without self-defeating and self-inhibiting feelings of anxiety, shame, and guilt. I try to live the life I want and respectfully assert my views in my personal and professional relationships. I think one example of this is the thesis of this chapter. I suspect my peers will disagree with the idea that REBT is a philosophy of life. In a professional world where evidence-based therapies are touted, calling REBT a philosophy of life, however accurate, may be viewed as undermining the claim that it is also an evidence-based psychotherapy. It may make it seem like taking this position brands the professional as a blind follower of Albert Ellis. I think that philosophers will question my view of REBT's metaphysics as a weak argument. In my younger years, fear would paralyze me, as I dreaded appearing foolish or deficient. However, REBT has helped me see that I do not need my point of view to be respected by significant others. I certainly want the respect, approval, and agreement of my colleagues, friends, and family, but I will choose to accept myself with or without their acceptance of the views I am putting forth in this chapter. I now believe that if others laugh at or criticize me or think poorly of me for my ideas or personal revelations and deficiencies, I do not have to be troubled by this form of rejection. I will choose not to reject myself even if others reject me or my views.

Before moving on, I should add that my unconditional self-acceptance also allows me to acknowledge my self-defeating tendency to occasionally anger myself and engage in impulsive behavior rooted in low discomfort tolerance. When I anger myself, I try to recognize this and transform my feelings into healthy ones that enable me to effectively respond to the interpersonal adversity I face.

Unconditional other-acceptance

The emotionally healthy person strives to accept other people unconditionally and see them as born mistake-makers. REBT philosophy acknowledges that it is useful to rate other people's behaviors. It recognizes that the individual is responsible for his actions but avoids a global judgment of the other person's value, whose conduct is the evaluation's focus. REBT philosophy holds that all standards for rating people as people are arbitrary, and therefore human worth cannot be objectively defined and validly determined. Using criteria, one can rate another person's behavior. REBT philosophy views all people as complex and continuously evolving beings, making total ratings invalid.

How do I implement unconditional other-acceptance in my life? I disagree with the intolerance of the American electorate. In my view, free speech is on the decline in the United States because political dissent is not tolerated. For example, years ago I told a friend and her partner a view I had on politics over dinner, hypothesizing a university professor would be open to intellectual discourse. I learned I was wrong in this assumption. That was the last dinner I had with that couple as they consistently rejected future dinner invitations, and they ended our friendship. I am sad that two women I had a friendship with would confuse a political view I shared with my value as a person and the importance of my friendship. I do not put these people down, but I think they hold rigid and extreme attitudes leading to intolerance of political dissent. I could anger myself by this act of intolerance. Instead, I harbor no ill will towards them and unconditionally accept them. They are fallible humans who have a perfect right to reject me and have a right to have intolerant views and act as they did towards me. I have come to appreciate not everyone unconditionally accepts other people who hold differing political opinions from their own. Since I value friendship and have been so strongly influenced by REBT's view of human fallibility, I hesitate to discuss politics and tolerate the discomfort of remaining silent when others discuss it. This is sad, but I accept that this is the case with fallible humans today.

I will add here that my ability to have unconditional other-acceptance has enabled me to learn from but not harbor any anger or ill-will towards four young men who threatened my life when I was in graduate school. In this incident, they assaulted me while I was walking to my parked car one night. As the incident unfolded, I was frightened for my life as I anticipated being shot or knifed to death. I was able to defend myself and live to tell the tale. I don't understand how a group of young men could perpetrate a violent unprovoked assault, but I accept that fallible humans do antisocial acts when they are young. I condemn the sin but accept those fallible, young men.

Self-responsibility for own emotional disturbance

In my view, REBT's emphasis on personal responsibility for one's emotional upset has a straightforward application to ethics which bolsters the argument that REBT qualifies as a philosophy of life. The Principle of Emotional Responsibility is the keystone of REBT. We hold ourselves accountable for our self-defeating emotional and behavioral reactions, even when others mistreat us. In REBT, there is no legitimacy to the idea of "righteous anger." Imagine a world where people lived according to this principle as a matter of routine. There certainly would be fewer interpersonal conflicts leading to arguments, violence, and looting. For example, in response to controversial incidents involving the police in multiple US cities and the related deaths of civilians in the months before the 2020 presidential election, the country witnessed widespread rioting, looting, and property destruction. In my view, a more positive result could have been achieved if people had adopted a philosophy of emotional responsibility and experienced healthy anger, which would lead to constructive, persistent, and powerful, peaceful protests. The destination of social justice can best be achieved through healthy anger and the implementation of REBT's Principle of Emotional Responsibility.

How do I apply the Principle of Emotional Responsibility in my life? I strive not to anger myself when people do uncivil things to me or in my neighborhood. In my community, the business district where I lease my private psychotherapy office and reside suffered widespread looting and property destruction due to civil unrest. One building blocks from my office was set on fire. Looting contributed to many businesses closing permanently, costing people their jobs. Tensions exist, and on four occasions over the past year young men have ridden bicycles towards me on the sidewalks of Philadelphia in an aggressive way. On these occasions, they have cycled quickly by me, traveling from behind to the point of startling me. It is difficult for me to conjure any other explanation than an effort to harass. I have also seen this done to women. This menacing behavior has occurred to my wife. I refuse to anger myself as I realize this will not stop such actions and only increase the probability of using poor judgment, which will endanger my safety. On one occasion, one of the young men turned his bicycle full circle and waited for me to pass on the other side of the street, perhaps looking to argue or fight. Had I not practiced REBT, I easily could have angered myself and walked across the street to confront him for his menacing behavior, but I accepted this would produce no useful outcome. Instead, I accepted what had occurred and was grateful I again was only startled instead of physically injured by this reckless behavior. I firmly believe my philosophical attitudes caused my self-helping feelings of self-protective concern and healthy anger. I also actively chose to feel sad and disappointed that people sometimes do this to me and others who live in my neighborhood. I feel sad for the business owners victimized by the riotous behavior and the people who have lost jobs, while at the same time condemning police misbehavior wherever it occurs. Nevertheless, thanks to my personal philosophy I will not anger or depress myself about these unfortunate events.

Unconditional life-acceptance

As an REBT psychologist, I encourage others to develop acceptance of life and strive to have some degree of happiness even when life is difficult and unfair. I see myself as a realist and do not believe a utopian existence can be achieved. Quoting Ellis, I actively teach patients that all paths have their advantages and disadvantages. I apply this concept when it comes to coping with the tradeoffs of living in Philadelphia. In a joint decision with my wife, we relocated ten years ago from Manhattan's Upper Eastside. We did this knowing Philadelphia is less to our liking, but the advantages of working at the University of Pennsylvania outweighed the disadvantages of living in Philadelphia.

When I look back on this decision, I believe I made the best one given our goals and values. Philadelphia has been very good to us. I have a better standard of living and enjoy my position at the University of Pennsylvania. I have the opportunity to train doctoral students in psychology and introduce them to REBT, which, sadly, is no longer taught in psychology postgraduate programs in the United States. My private practice is busy. Through my affiliation with the University of Pennsylvania, I have had the chance to perform in the role of a subject matter expert on a project that aims to teach CBT skills to the US Navy's enlisted sailors. However, ten years on, I am more aware of how Philadelphia is a much less desirable place to live in than Manhattan.

I miss living in Manhattan. The streets and sidewalks of Philadelphia are poorly maintained. There is considerably more litter on the streets. There is less to see and to do. The transportation system is not as useful and considerably more limited than the New York City subway system and the associated suburban railroads of Long Island and Connecticut. I regularly remind myself, my wife, and my patients that there are no ideal solutions in life. I remind myself that this is my home, and I can choose to live happily, nonetheless. I keep in mind that I will not get these years back at the end of my life. I strive to live fully where I now reside so that I have no regret on my death bed that "I could have been happy in Philadelphia if only I had accepted the good with the bad during those years." In REBT, we see life as a mix of good, bad, and neutral parts. This view of life applies to my life in Philadelphia, and I unconditionally accept my life here and accept Philadelphia warts and all.

Another way I practice unconditional life-acceptance is my choosing to feel happy despite being denied children. Being unable to have my own biological family was a great disappointment to my wife and me. However, I can honestly say that I have learned to see the good in the bad. I wish I had been blessed with a child or two I could have taught REBT philosophy to and enjoyed a great deal of laughter with over the years. However, thanks to unconditional life-acceptance, I can also see that there are clear advantages in not having children. I do acknowledge that not having had children of my own has contributed to a deficit in experiential knowledge, which I could have used as a psychologist. I share this great disappointment with my patients in the service of showing them that, with REBT philosophy, they too can have some degree of happiness despite life's great disappointments.

Calculated risk-taking

REBT teaches that the emotionally healthy person accepts life's uncertainty and is capable of taking calculated risks to maximize their pleasure in life and achieve self-selected goals. They take these risks with a full appreciation of the possible benefits and potential losses that may ensue. When risk-taking fails to achieve the desired outcome, the emotionally healthy person relies on unconditional self-acceptance, unconditional life-acceptance, and their ability to manage their emotional reactions to tolerate the consequences of their actions and the disappointments of life. What sorts of calculated risks have I taken? As mentioned previously, I see my choice of profession, spouse, and decision to move to Philadelphia all as past calculated risks. Two additional calculated risks involved an apartment and an office I decided to rent and the impact on my personal finances if the risks did not pan out in my favor.

When my wife and I married, we lived in an apartment she owned in Brooklyn. We both preferred living in Manhattan and ultimately found an incredible Manhattan apartment. We immediately recognized how lucky we were to have located a particular apartment on the elegant Upper Eastside of Manhattan three blocks east of the original Albert Ellis Institute. We appreciated this particular apartment because we knew the Manhattan rental market. However, there was a risk in signing a lease on this apartment while it was still available, as we did not have a prospective renter to occupy my wife's apartment in Brooklyn, which carried a monthly mortgage. Our reserve cash funds would only cover the mortgage for three months. Without a renter at the ready for our Brooklyn apartment, signing a lease on the Manhattan apartment was a calculated financial risk. However, because of the high discomfort tolerance I had used for getting to know the Manhattan rental market, I knew not to relinquish the opportunity with this exceptional apartment. Signing the lease was a risk worth taking. REBT philosophy figured into my reasoning as I did not "absolutely need a guarantee" that my gamble would pay off. I was concerned, but not anxious. I assumed I could work to find a reliable renter for the Brooklyn apartment within three months. In the end, I found a renter, and my calculated risk paid off. If I had let that incredible apartment go because I could not tolerate risk, I have no doubt I would have later regretted playing things safe and passing on the apartment due to fear of financial failure.

I took a similar risk while upgrading my professional office and signing a five-year lease. Once again, my high discomfort tolerance paid off, and with a great deal of effort I found an incredible office that met all my requirements. However, it was more expensive than I had ever paid in terms of monthly rent and I would have to expand my hours and raise my fee to make it sufficiently profitable. I sat with my Excel spreadsheet, made what I considered reasonable assumptions, and made the five-year commitment. I can honestly say this calculated risk paid off well beyond my expectations. Again it helped me that REBT teaches that, to live life well, one had better be capable of tolerating uncertainty instead of demanding that all risks would pan out. My uncertainty tolerance enabled me to sign the lease and profit from the calculated risk I took.

Long-term hedonism

REBT encourages people to maximize pleasure in life and live for a healthy balance between the moment's pleasures and the greater pleasure one would derive by delaying gratification. I have shifted my lifestyle from one that was oriented towards short-term hedonism to one that maximizes pleasure through long-term hedonism. The first example of this is my choice of professions. Earning my doctorate in psychology took considerable effort over no less than five years beyond undergraduate and master's level training. When I chose to enter psychotherapy by earning a doctorate, I was delaying gratification by pursuing the highest level of training. I could have stopped my education and practiced as a master's level psychotherapist. However, I took the longer path through the demanding scientist-practitioner doctoral training program to maximize my long-term pleasure.

However, my commitment did not stop with my choice to pursue extensive postgraduate training. During this period, I also decided that I had better heed Ellis's advice and practice what I preached (Ellis, 2007). I decided that, to evolve into the most effective REBT psychotherapist I could become, I had to overcome my addiction to cannabis. I also became aware that to overcome this self-defeating habit I would have to give up sporadic binge drinking that inevitably seemed to be linked with a relapse in smoking cannabis or lead to foolish, self-defeating behavior. Giving up this pleasure while living in Manhattan was hard to do. I stayed with this goal because I wanted to be a very effective REBT psychotherapist. At this time, I used both REBT and exercise to help me evolve into a long-term hedonist. It was time to walk the talk of REBT philosophy. I eventually ran my first New York City marathon and used long-distance running as a coping method. Running every day gave my life structure, helped me relax, and enabled me to meet interesting people and, most importantly, cope with a chronic low-grade depression that seems to be largely biologically based. My first New York City marathon led to my second NYC marathon, culminating in a streak of thirteen before an injury ended my career. However, those thirteen marathons served to help me transition from short-term to long-term hedonism.

For 31 years, I have abstained from all types of smoking and live an alcohol-free life. Consistent with REBT philosophy, I have never labeled myself anything other than a fallible human. I acknowledged that I once engaged in self-defeating substance abuse and now cope with my problems rationally and enjoy life more fully without the highs and lows of substance use. I now have added Wellbutrin and a pharmaceutical-grade B complex designed explicitly for post-partum depression. These help me perform at my very best and enjoy life to the fullest. Marathons, REBT, and psychotropics interact synergistically and have allowed me to go from short-term hedonism to a more satisfying and authentic long-term hedonistic lifestyle. Since I have made this transition, I have a new goal. I never ask a patient to do a homework assignment that I would consider too hard, too inconvenient, or too uncomfortable to do. These homework assignments include counting calories to maintain a healthy weight, structuring my life to get sufficient sleep, taking calculated risks, and getting out of my comfort zone by writing books and chapter articles. I am willing to tolerate the discomfort of doing what is best in the long run despite the short-term pain involved. As I tell my patients, "I assume I do not have to feel like doing a task in order to do it when it is the right time to do it." This assumption generally helps me stay true to the REBT philosophy of long-term hedonism.

Healthy sense of humor

Ellis always taught that the emotionally healthy person maintains a healthy sense of humor by not taking themselves, others, or life itself too seriously or not seriously enough. The emotionally healthy person has concerns but does not cross the line into over-seriousness associated with emotional disturbance. In my life, I have, at times, been too serious in my approach to life. My seriousness was on display when I attended the oldest Quaker school in the world founded by William Penn in the city of Philadelphia. I was fortunate to attend such a highly competitive college preparatory school. While there I was a varsity athlete in two sports for all four of my high school years. I was young and determined to make the most of my education, to excel at athletics, but did not have a good sense of humor. I was in continuous motion and always studying. I was chronically sleep-deprived due to regularly studying late into the night. I was prone to depression when I failed or fell short of my high standards. Falling short did not happen too often, which was fortunate as I disturbed myself badly when I did. Failure on the athletic field was especially difficult for me to accept. I also was a procrastinator at times when it came to writing papers.

During my high school years, I discovered that my thinking exerted a profound influence on my emotional reactions and became interested in psychology. While progressing through my undergraduate degree at the University of Pennsylvania, I learned to loosen up, enjoy myself a bit, and not take life so seriously. I was learning Beck's Cognitive Therapy and yet to learn about REBT. At this time self-esteem was important to me and I was certainly living my life to prove myself instead of living it to enjoy myself. When I was deeply exposed to REBT and Albert Ellis in graduate school at Hofstra University, his philosophy taught me how to laugh at what I did and stop trying to save the world. As a psychologist in training, I was interested in developing my career and becoming known. REBT helped me become a long-term hedonist, but I also had to learn I could not and did not have to save the world. I came to understand the value of doing better but not being better or lesser than other people.

I now honestly believe I do not take myself or my life too seriously. I continue to strive for excellence in nearly all that I do, especially my work as an REBT psychologist. I try to have fun with my students when teaching REBT and use humor as part of my work with patients to help them see that when they make demands leading to emotional disturbance, they inevitably are taking things too seriously. Laughing for me is a gift from nature, a healthy and natural drug, and I enjoy laughing throughout the day in a good-natured and appropriate way, as much as I possibly can. I often say that I hope to die with a deep sense of unconditional self-acceptance as I review my life in my final hours. It would be preferable to live my last minutes laughing healthily with my wife if she were still alive or some other dear friend close at hand. To die laughing in a healthy way is one way of having some leverage over death as I take my final breath.

Semantic precision

As I have practiced REBT over my thirty-year career, I have grown increasingly interested in REBT's roots and how Ellis weaved it together from ancient and modern philosophy. To this end, I have begun to study both Alfred Korzybski's General Semantics theory and Stoicism, Epicureanism, and to a lesser extent Aristotelianism and Buddhism. I was surprised how closely REBT parallels General Semantics Theory and have committed to semantic precision. I do not go as far as to speak in e-prime, although one day I may; I must admit it fascinates me. As stated earlier, Ellis argued the best REBT psychotherapists practice what they preach, and for me that involves striving to implement semantic precision when thinking and speaking. Although I grew up in a household where other people were too often labeled, I honestly can say my REBT philosophy includes my commitment not to label people and overgeneralize when they misbehave. I have learned that the Stoics advocated we discipline our minds through morning and evening meditation and negative visualization. In addition to practicing these Stoic meditative exercises, I strive to discipline my mind to think in a semantically precise way. I want to reap the benefits of this way of thinking, model it for my patients, and not open myself to the charge of hypocrisy when I challenge my patients and students to embrace this way of thinking about themselves, others, and the world in which we live.

Areas where I struggle to implement REBT effectively or consistently

Reader, please take note that, despite practicing REBT for over thirty years, there are areas in my life where I have difficulty implementing it effectively or consistently. I hope to impress upon the reader that I honestly believe that my struggle to implement this philosophy will continue until my final hour. I do not doubt that my effort towards unconditional self-acceptance and unconditional life-acceptance will be ongoing until the moment of my last breath. Furthermore, I see discomfort tolerance as something I possess in differing degrees across my life's many domains. Although I may demonstrate very high discomfort tolerance in some areas of life, I recognize areas where I exercise low discomfort tolerance and wish to improve. Due to space limitations, I will restrict my discussion to three categories where I still struggle to implement REBT philosophy.

Struggling with anxiety due to a tendency to awfulize

My wife and I have grown our financial assets over the years by living within our means and seeking and consistently following independent, expert financial advice from the outset of our marriage some twenty-six years ago. However, I often find I experience significant stress and anxiety when I have to buy, sell, or move large sums of money between funds, accounts, and financial institutions. I recently moved a sizable retirement account from one institution to another. I made myself very stressed and anxious by demanding that I not implement the transfer improperly and inadvertently buy the wrong mutual funds. I checked with a fund representative multiple times before I hit the submit button and was quite stressed before, during, and after authorizing these transactions. I acted as if it would be the end of the world if I bought the wrong bond funds even though the mistake would have been reversible after the accounts settled. However, I still appear to hold the rigid attitude that "I have to be an efficient investor" and "Because my financial well-being is important, I, therefore, have to maximize returns by avoiding asset deployment mistakes." Due to this idea, I sometimes irrationally reason that to choose the wrong funds would be awful, terrible, and the end of the world.

Struggling with discomfort anxiety

Although I no longer consume alcohol and honestly have no struggle whatsoever doing this despite it being at the ready in my home for guests, I cannot say the same when it comes to food consumption. Due to my family background, I am at significant risk for Type 2 diabetes. To address this, I am vigilant to maintain a healthy weight by consistently adhering to a low-fat, high-fiber diet. My wife is a gourmet home cook who supports me by producing wholesome and delicious meals in small portion sizes. The struggle occurs when there is some amount of food that may be extra despite her best efforts. I joke that I am like a fish and will eat what is available even though I am no longer hungry. I seem to hold the attitude, "If there is delicious food left over, I have to consume it, and it is unbearable not to do so." Fortunately, she has worked closely with me on this weakness by consistently preparing small servings of food. Still, I struggle nonetheless because occasionally she will not always finish her portion of dinner. Her unfinished food sits for me to drool over and then experience the urge to eat. Too often, I yield to the desire. I consistently maintain a healthy weight well within the body mass index limits. Still, it would be far better to avoid eating her leftovers or any small extra amount she inadvertently has prepared. Despite my healthy weight, a few more pounds lost would probably yield even more insurance against my health risks. Plato said, "For a man to conquer himself is the first and noblest of all victories." If I were to cultivate the discomfort tolerance to consistently resist the urge to eat leftover food when I have already consumed a healthy amount, it would be gratifying for me to achieve.

A second area of having a low tolerance for discomfort is filing in the digital world and the real world. I am prone to rushing to do my work and often quickly stick a document in a new file folder rather than finding an appropriate existing file folder. This impulsive behavior leads to an electronic file folder structure that is rather long. The consequence of this file folder structure is that it makes efficiently locating important files difficult. I sometimes rush to file a document because I hold the attitude that "I have to move on and get things done quickly – it's too hard to find an existing folder to store this piece of information." I will sometimes quickly stick a paper in a drawer in real life rather than carefully file it in order to make it easy to locate in the future.

A third and crucial area of discomfort intolerance has to do with overall personal efficiency and working tensely. I have always appreciated that time is not an elastic resource and desired to remain focused and not procrastinate throughout the day. I sometimes will notice undesirable variability in my efficiency during my professional workday. Furthermore, I am often rushing to get more done as if I could finish the unending list of things I find to do. When I have a free hour or two, I sometimes do not get down to business doing an uncomfortable task as quickly as I theoretically could. Sometimes I am distracted by relatively low priority tasks. My efficiency may also suffer when I am too exacting about how well or thoroughly I might do a relatively unimportant task. My goal is to maximize my professional output while being relaxed and efficient, and I believe there is still room for improvement in this highly valued area of my life. A personal goal is to produce more material disseminating REBT. Greater efficiency with less inner tension throughout the workweek would serve me well.

Struggling with people rating

As the reader can guess by this point, I have a strong preference for REBT as an approach to psychotherapy and a personal philosophy of life. I do not delude myself into believing it is perfect, and all my patients will do well with it. No system of psychotherapy is perfect and can work with everyone. Ellis may have been a genius, but it does not mean he created a therapy or philosophy which cannot be improved. He was a human, and although REBT is excellent therapy, it remains an imperfect product of his life's mission. However, REBT profoundly resonates with me and will be the only therapeutic approach that I am comfortable failing with when attempting to help a patient who is suffering. Succeeding with my patients is very important to me. When I fall short as a psychotherapist, I want to do so with what seems to be an efficient, effective, and broadly applicable therapy that can produce enduring effects. I want to fail only with my best effort. Over my career, I have remained an adherent to the REBT teachings Ellis modeled and taught because I have not found a better approach to doing what I do for a living and a philosophy of life. Therefore, I need to guard against rating and downgrading colleagues who do not appreciate this form of therapy or philosophy. More specifically, I greatly value teaching my patients self-direction and emotional responsibility and doing this efficiently. I sometimes struggle not to cross the line into thinking rigidly that my colleagues should also emphasize the teaching of self-direction, emotional responsibility for one's emotional upset, rational thinking, and therapeutic efficiency to the extent that I do. I sometimes struggle to understand how other professionals can adopt therapeutic systems that do not embrace the other elements I have discussed throughout this chapter. I have difficulty understanding how my colleagues could not come to appreciate the liberating power REBT offers patients and therapists alike. I want to remain faithful to my philosophy and challenge the idea that others must share the therapeutic enlightenment I have achieved. I do not wish to become an REBT fascist who does not genuinely embrace unconditional acceptance of those who do not understand and appreciate the many advantages of Rational Emotive Behavior Therapy.

Advantages of REBT as a philosophy of life

I hope by this point the reader will agree that REBT qualifies as a philosophy of life because it has both metaphysics and ethics. Unlike other cognitive-behavior therapies, it is more than a collection of therapeutic techniques tied together by a case conceptualization and applied to DSM diagnoses. REBT can be used in this way because it was created in a real-world clinic to address clinical disorders and problems of daily living. However, as Ellis proceeded, he went from psychotherapy to philosophy when he articulated the eleven elements of well-being addressed above. Furthermore, I believe there are clear advantages to seeing REBT as more than merely a psychotherapy that one employs during one's professional work to help others. When the practitioner embodies REBT and embraces it as a philosophy, as Ellis himself did, they improve their therapeutic potency by being an authentic representative of the philosophy they are teaching. This position raises the standard the psychotherapist aspires to. In my view, patients study the psychotherapist as much as the psychotherapist examines the patient. I suspect there is a nonspecific factor that comes into play by this display of authenticity. However, beyond authenticity, embodying the theory as a philosophy of life gives the psychotherapist greater empathy for their patients' struggles to implement REBT. This authenticity and empathy probably add to the practitioner's therapeutic potency. I always tell my students and patients that REBT asks a great deal of both the psychotherapist and the patient. To develop a genuine sense of unconditional self, unconditional other, and unconditional life acceptance is damn hard. Psychotherapists and their patients are fallible humans. Holding flexible and nonextreme attitudes towards the most challenging aspects of life, including one's health and ultimate demise, is not always easy to do. The payoff of disciplining one's mind with REBT's philosophy is equal to the degree of difficulty and importance of the adversity faced. REBT is the CBT of choice when your worst nightmare has occurred or may very well happen. During the current Covid-19 pandemic, the philosophy has served me well and enabled me to remain emotionally strong and to help my patients by reminding them that the pandemic, in an absolute sense, should be happening because it is happening, that although it is bad, things can always be worse, that they can bear the discomfort they feel for however long the pandemic exists, and that life is not totally bad. By embracing REBT philosophy, I have managed to have some degree of happiness during the pandemic. I encourage my patients to strive to live healthily and to some extent happily during the pandemic simply because when it is over, none of us will get a refund for the year or years we lived under the restrictions necessitated by the pandemic. Time only goes forward. Seeing REBT as a philosophy has given me the strength to control what is under my control. It helps me to accept all that is well beyond my control while maintaining my sense of humor about it all.

By seeing REBT as a philosophy, I derive greater enjoyment and meaning from my work. My thirty-plus sessions each week are a labor of love. As a psychologist, adjunct professor, clinical trainer, and psychotherapist, my work is not a job but a mission to share a philosophy I believe in, love, and use every day. I hope to disseminate this powerful philosophy to the broadest possible audience. In my view, if more people knew of this philosophy, the world would be a very different place with considerably less suffering. There would be less hostility in human affairs at all levels, from families to groups, to possibly even nations. I doubt the entire world will ever adopt REBT's philosophy and embrace it as I have, as it certainly is not the only path to happiness, serenity, and meaning available to people. I also think it requires a great deal from humans and, due to our biological predisposition to discomfort disturbance, REBT will ask for too much effort for many people. I am not delusional and think it is perfect and should not continue to be refined by precise and scientific thinking. I continue to advocate for the empirical examination of it in clinical practice. However, I believe REBT psychotherapists who embody it as a philosophy will not only be better role models to their patients and enhance their therapy, but will also be happier and healthier practitioners. These practitioners will stand apart from other CBT psychotherapists who do not have a psychotherapeutic system that rests upon an underlying philosophy of life.

Potential disadvantages of REBT as a philosophy of life

As Ellis said, every course of action has its advantages and disadvantages. What are the disadvantages of seeing REBT as a philosophy? There is the risk that its scientific outlook and emphasis on empirical verification could erode. If zealous adopters and practitioners of REBT begin to demand that others adopt it and see it as a perfect path and the only way of proceeding through the messy journey of life, there is the risk of hypocrisy. However, as long as the practitioners and adopters of this philosophy and psychotherapy stay true to the theory of nondogmatic thinking, I believe most of the disadvantages can be minimized. As a philosophy of life and as psychotherapy, REBT can make a resurgence in the world of the 21st century and thereby help humans reduce pain and increase their pleasure and meaning as they inevitably stumble through their lives.

Note

1 I have no conflicts of interest to disclose. Correspondence concerning this chapter should be addressed to Walter J. Matweychuk.

References

Dryden, W. (2013). *Rationality and pluralism: The selected works of Windy Dryden.* London: Routledge, Taylor & Francis Group.

Dryden, W. (2015). *Rational emotive behavior therapy: Distinctive features.* 2nd edition. Hove, East Sussex: Routledge.

Ellis, A. (1996). *Reason and emotion in psychotherapy: A comprehensive method of treating human disturbances.* 2nd edition. New York, NY: Citadel.

Ellis, A. (2004). *Rational emotive behavior therapy: It works for me – it can work for you.* Amherst, NY: Prometheus Books.

Ellis, A. (2007). *Overcoming resistance: A rational emotive behavior therapy integrated approach.* New York, NY: Springer.

Ellis, A., & Becker, I. (1982). *Guide to personal happiness.* Hollywood, CA: Wilshire Bk, LA.

Ellis, A., & Dryden, W. (2007). *The practice of rational emotive behavior therapy.* New York, NY: Springer.

Pigliucci, M., Cleary, S., & Kaufman, D. (2020). *How to live a good life: A guide to choosing the right personal philosophy.* New York, NY: Vintage Books/Penguin Random House LLC.

Velten, E.C. (2007). *Under the influence: Reflections of Albert Ellis in the work of others.* Tucson, AZ: See Sharp Press.

Walen, S.R., DiGiuseppe, R., & Dryden, W. (1992). *Practitioner's guide to rational-emotive therapy.* Oxford: Oxford University Press.

Epilogue

Chapter 10

Rational Emotive Behavior Therapy

Past, present, and future in the CBT community

Arthur Freeman[1]

This chapter offers an integrative and affectionate perspective on the past, present, and future of Rational Emotive Behavior Therapy (REBT) within the cognitive-behavioral therapies (CBT) community. It starts by describing the roots of REBT and the challenges that it faced over time with respect to its identity. The present of REBT is discussed next, by mentioning the pioneers of REBT that advanced the field and emphasizing the perils brought by reinventing the wheel, together with potential reasons for this practice. In the end, the chapter includes important lessons for the future and for the survival of REBT, many of which are embedded in stories and metaphors.

The roots of Rational Emotive Behavior Therapy

Over 40 years ago, Michael Mahoney (1977) called Cognitive-Behavior Therapy (CBT) "the barbarians at the gates" banging on the door of the psychotherapy establishment and psychodynamic therapy in particular. We were demanding entrance and were being denied by the forces/persons within. Four decades later, we have become the guardians of the gates and CBT has become the gold standard for psychotherapy around the world.

This happened two decades after Albert Ellis had introduced and promoted his revolutionary treatment of Rational Therapy (RT; Ellis, 1962). He, and his early students and co-workers, started a journey that has brought us to today, in Cluj-Napoca, through the modifications of RT to Rational Emotive Therapy (RET) and Rational Emotive Behavior Therapy (REBT). This willingness (or at times hard-fought unwillingness) to modify our model was the beginning of our path of development and growth.

Nowadays, there are many terms within the CBT community that could be called Branding Terms (amongst other terms), such as those used historically: Rational Therapy, Rational Emotive Therapy, Rational Emotive Behavior Therapy, Rational Behavior Modification, Cognitive Therapy, Cognitive-Behavioral Therapy, Cognitive-Behavioral Modification, Multi-Modal Therapy, Dialectical Behavioral Therapy, Acceptance and

DOI: 10.4324/9781003081593-14

Commitment Therapy. So we can look at CBT as a collection of brand names. These treatment branding titles have, by and large, fallen away over the years so that CBT has become the generic term for what we do. Should we maintain them? Should REBT continue to label and brand itself as REBT or under a more general term such as CBT? How can we preserve our identity amidst all of the changes and developments? In fact, should we try to maintain our REBT identity?

It is clear that REBT has its own attributes such as that it is a method of psychotherapy, a mode of thinking about oneself, the world, and the future, and a model of approaching life's challenges, and a multimodal intervention that encompasses cognition, behavior, emotion, temperament, culture, and outreach.

REBT in the present

Many promoters of new approaches in psychotherapies do not acknowledge and recognize the other models/philosophies that informed their progress. Many students, however, these days are not familiar with previous contributions to the field. What I find troubling is that this can happen also to people who make great contributions to the field but do not acknowledge theories that they integrate in their work. Jeffrey Young was interviewed and asked about the similarities with the work of Adler and he answered that he is not familiar with that. Why not? Many of you are familiar with the book by David Burns (1980) called *Feeling Good*, which has sold six million copies. David Burns worked with Dr. Beck. Its publisher implied that he founded CT and when he was asked about this, he said that he cannot control what others write. Albert Ellis always called himself an Adlerian, and acknowledged the influence that this approach had on his theory.

Thus, we can look around and see where we are. But where did we come from? The following list cannot be comprehensive but provides the names of persons/models which need to be and hopefully are familiar to any CBT practitioner and can be called "heroes" of REBT/CBT:

- Epictetus – Stoicism
- Alfred Adler – Individual Psychology
- Shoma Morita – Morita Therapy
- Joseph Wolpe – Systematic desensitization
- Albert Ellis – REBT
- George Kelly – Personal Construct Therapy
- Victor Frankl – Logotherapy
- Aaron T. Beck – Cognitive Therapy
- Maxie Maultsby – Rational Behavior Modification
- Michael Mahoney – Constructivist Cognitive Behavior Therapy

- Arnold Lazarus – Multimodal Therapy
- Donald Meichenbaum – Cognitive Behavior Modification
- Marsha Linehan – Dialectical Behavior Therapy
- Steven Hayes – Acceptance and Commitment Therapy
- Thomas D'Zuirilla/Arthur and Christine Nezu – Problem-Solving Training
- Martin Seligman – Positive Psychology
- Paul Gilbert – Compassion-Focused Cognitive Therapy
- Zindel Segal – Mindfulness-Based Cognitive Therapy
- Daniel David – Technology-Based REBT
- Jeffrey Young – Schema Therapy
- Windy Dryden – Single Session REBT, major historian (the most published author in REBT/CBT in the world)
- Ann Vernon – School-Based REBT
- Kristine Doyle – Eating Disorders
- Ray DiGiuseppe – Anger Management
- Oana David – Cognitive Behavioral Coaching
- Tullio Scrimali – Neuroscience-Based Cognitive Therapy

Each of these pioneers of REBT added a new twist, or addressed a hitherto untouched problem, issue, treatment venue, field extension, patient population, treatment context, or cultural adaptation.

Too often, the "new developments" in REBT and CBT, more broadly, have been renamed or repackaged iterations of what could easily be found in the extant literature. I recall an experience with Ray DiGiuseppe at a meeting of the Association for Advancement of Behavior Therapy (now ABCT). It was a crowded auditorium and we were standing in the back listening to the presidential address; as the outgoing president offered his comments and vision for the future, Ray became more and more upset. When I asked Ray what was upsetting him, he said, "Al said all of these things years ago and now someone else has claimed credit without a single historical attribution or citation!" We find that there are always people that keep reinventing the wheel. Why does this happen in the therapeutic field? Reasons can be related to many factors, among which are: therapeutic narcissism of the person, ignorance of the theoretical, philosophical, contextual content and overall goals of a treatment model, the fact that the person is only educated in a unimodal model, or is working within a rigid model (e.g., reusing old terms).

Reticence toward the new paradigms is common to the psychotherapeutic field, but it is essential that we acknowledge the importance of inclusion and diversity and we learn from our past. We need to learn that although the therapists having a behavioral approach first rejected the cognitive therapy paradigm, latterly it was integrated and thus we witnessed, for example, the development from the European Association of Behavioral Therapy (EABT) to the European Association of Behavioral and Cognitive Therapy (EABCT), and from the American Association of Behavioral Therapy (AABT) to the American Association for Behavioral and Cognitive Therapies (ABCT).

The number of countries and cultures represented at this Fourth Congress of REBT in Cluj-Napoca evidences the growth and importance of an international REBT emphasis. And this is key since we are an international movement and not a splinter group and REBT needs to view itself in this way. Thus, we need to find venues for sharing REBT.

However, the problem is that we often make few attempts to bring new, younger, creative people into our group. It is essential for us to reach out to attract new members to our REBT groups. We can do this through various venues, such as dedicated journals, websites, workshops, podcasts, or local, regional, national, and international meetings. We could put together a task force for applications of REBT. A couple of years ago I published a book about CBT for social workers. It was an excellent book but did not sell well since REBT is not popular among social workers.

Lessons for the future and for the survival of REBT

Many of the pioneers have passed on, and their places have been taken by their students and now by the "grandchildren" of the founders. We need to think about how we build continuity.

What offers us the gift of continuity? If it was the personality of the founder that provided the glue that held us together, the model may experience an erosion and remain limited. There will always be the "true believers" who may want to limit or avoid any advances or development of the model to preserve the perceived authenticity of the model. My experience is that I studied at the Alfred Adler Institute in New York in 1966. We had a supervision group and one of the members suggested why don't we try this. There was a member in the group who studied with Adler in Vienna and she said no, no, no! Adler would not have approved! She wanted to keep Adlerian psychology where it was in the 1930s. Moreover, if you want to apply to present at a North American Society of Adlerian Psychotherapy Congress, a requirement is that you have presented at the previous congress. So they are talking to themselves and this way the group is becoming older and smaller.

The main lessons to be learned and that Adler would teach are:

1. Be courageous. When you are a child and you try to walk, you fall. And you need to get up and try again. We all did this.
2. Be flexible. This does not mean to twist and turn to the demands of others but learning what is new and including that in what we do – for example, the advances in neurosciences and in technology and how do we include them in what we do.

3. Be willing to be vulnerable. To say something publicly, make statements and defend what we believe in.
4. Be willing to be fallible and make mistakes.
5. Be creative. Some of the most creative people in this field are at this congress.
6. Be proactive. We cannot simply react but be proactive to what the field needs.
7. Address community needs. We need to adapt to what the current needs are.
8. Be culturally sensitive and aware.
9. Emphasize the importance of empirical support for REBT/CBT. We need to focus on empirical support for what we do.

I love books. I have lots and lots of books. And I cannot resist going into a bookstore and looking at the shelves of old books and always finding something of interest. Many years ago, I entered a bookstore and I found a book called *Peony*, written by Pearl S. Buck (1948), Nobel Prize winner. I took it home and I have re-read it over the years and I have thought of it in connection to this presentation. Let me tell you about Peony:

> The city of Kaifeng in China was a center for Jewish habitation in the 19th century. Many Jewish merchants and their families were successful and lived and worked there upon the famed Silk Route. Consistent with their tradition, the Jewish merchants built a large and beautiful synagogue as a center for their worship and community. The story of Peony is about a Jewish family and their life and interactions with the local Chinese population. It is a story of interchange of ideas and beliefs and also the intermarriage of the Jewish families into the majority Chinese culture until the core of the beliefs of the Jews were lost to sight by all but the most observant. Peony was originally a bond-maiden in the house of David Ben Ezra. In her later years she became the abbess of the monastery. Reflective in her senior years, she pondered her life and reflected on what she had done and not done in her life and the rightness of her actions. She concluded that nothing is lost and they all live again and forever, with their spirit reborn in every new generation.

Is this the fate of the revolutionary and visionary work of Albert Ellis? Will his ideas be subsumed, interwoven, renamed, imitated, stolen, or repurposed into the ideas and theories and therapies of countless other models? Or, will the ideas of REBT stand firm and well used into the growth and development by his students (many of us), and the numbers of generations to follow us. Not CBT generically, but REBT most specifically.

Conclusions

We need to learn and teach the work of our founders and pioneers. We need to not try to re-invent the wheel, but learn to better use and develop the wheels that we have. Be proud to stand on the shoulders of giants. This lofty perspective allows us to view the past, experience the present, and move REBT to the future. And this is, I think, our model; we look to the past for information, we look to the future so we know where we are going but we stay focused in the present.

As you know, Ellis wrote many songs and in his honor I wrote a song. As a shame attack I challenge you to sing with me. I used the old song melody "Oh Susana" and I called it "A musical tribute to Albert Ellis":

Oh, he came from New York City with Sigmund in his sights.
He started small but ended up at fantastic heights.
Oh, Al Ellis, there is so much we could say.
For all that you have given us, we honor you today.

He spoke of musturbation, of should and musts and oughts.
He taught us how to recognize our irrational thoughts.
Oh, Al Ellis, there is so much we could say.
For all that you have given us, we honor you today.

He talked the talk and walked the walk and pioneered the way
For us to practice CBT, which flourishes today.
Oh, Al Ellis, there is so much we could say.
For all that you have given us, we honor you today.

He shocked us with his style, a therapeutic Puck
Who peppered his discussions with words like sheet and f**k.
Oh, Al Ellis, there is so much we could say.
For all that you have given us, we honor you today.

He offered change in therapy, a philosophic view
Taught throughout the world today from him to all of you.
Oh, Al Ellis, there is so much we could say.
For all that you have given us, we honor you today.

Now you're gone, we honor you. What else would you expect?
We send you this last message. To Al with big respect.
[Big ending:]
Oh, Al Ellis, there is so much we could say.
For all that you have given us, we honor you today.

Note

1 In memoriam of Professor Arthur Freeman, prepared by Oana David, Ph.D., and Daniel David, Ph.D., based on the keynote presented by Arthur Freeman, Ed.D., at the Fourth International Congress of Rational Emotive Behavior Therapy, September 13–15, 2019, in Cluj-Napoca, Transylvania, Romania.

References

Buck, P.S. (1948). *Peony*. New York: The John Day Company.

Burns, D.D. (1980). *Feeling good: The new mood therapy*. New York: Wm. Morrow and Co.

Ellis, A. (1962). *Reason and emotion in psychotherapy*. New York: Lyle Stuart.

Mahoney, M.J. (1977). Personal science: A cognitive learning therapy. In A. Ellis & R. Grieger (Eds.), *Handbook of rational-emotive therapy* (pp. 352–368). New York: Springer.

Postscript

Art Freeman, Ed.D. (1942–2020), a eulogy

Mark Gilson

My history with Art goes back to the early 1980s when I was a fellow at the Center for Cognitive Therapy at Penn and Art was Tim Beck's clinical director. At that time, different members of the Center supervised and taught. Art was just getting his bearings as a speaker and an author. Most noticeable was that, unlike many of the faculty and members of the Center in Philadelphia, Art took great delight in making people laugh as they learned. He would tell stories that usually had a level of absurdity that would lead us to break up and ultimately get the point he was trying to make. He used Borscht belt comedians combined with TV evangelists as models. The Jewishness was always there and it made me happy. In our last trip with him and his partner Rosie to Romania for the REBT Congress in 2019, Art was the only presenter who got a standing ovation because that is what he does. He got a crowd of serious mental health professionals acting uncharacteristically joyful by being both silly and engaging.

Art was always someone with more ideas than he could possibly handle, and if you were listening to what he proposed, you might find yourself part of a book project, a presenter at a conference, or some other big idea. I owed so much to his generosity. I kept thinking, as he was dying, that when he got to heaven, he would ask other deceased psychologists and students to work on a book about "Cognitive Therapy for Dying and the Afterlife."

Make no mistake. Art wanted to live. He wanted to travel and meet people like he had done for the past forty years, going to almost every country in the world. He loved to present on cognitive therapy and to establish contacts with mental health professionals everywhere you can imagine. He lived to network with other professionals. He was generous and felt good when he was part of what led others to thrive and succeed. I know this personally because when I left Philadelphia, he pushed me to do something more than take a job for someone else. His idea for a training program looked impossible for one person to do, but he kept saying I had the abilities. He helped me start a professional training program in 1985. I am now trying to model Art and pass it on to younger psychologists who are taking the helm.

DOI: 10.4324/9781003081593-15

I started to reflect on the last three and a half years. Art met his partner Rosie before he was diagnosed with cancer. Soon after they met, both had a weird trip to Russia where the Russians detained him for three weeks for an expired visa until he finally came home to NYC. He and Rosie were quickly falling for each other, and then came the devastating Sloan Kettering diagnosis of pancreatic cancer. There has to be a Putin joke in here somewhere, but that would be tasteless. Back in 2017 the prognosis was dire, but Art was determined to fight. There were many problems that individually would have taken any of us down for the count. The short list is: pancreatic cancer, broken neck, Covid-19, liver cancer, open heart surgery, and sepsis. Like I said, Art loved life and he was determined to live it. Art liked using *Fiddler on the Roof* to teach lessons in finding alternative interpretations. He would use the scene where Tevye kept trying to decide about giving his blessing for his daughter's marriage that did not follow tradition. On one hand, on the other hand, and back and forth Tevye went until he could no longer think of an alternative and there was no other hand. The diseases got in the way, but Art kept finding his way around the maladies and kept finding the other hand that kept him alive a little longer. It went on till the only alternative was one he could no longer control

Art had a weakness that could have killed him without any of the diseases. He kept falling for women and was blind to any problems they posed for him and he for them once he fell in love. We saw him through numerous marriages and girlfriends, sometimes occurring concurrently. Whenever he did fall in love, he seemed to want to have yet another marriage. The delight was how deeply he felt for the women he cared about. I don't remember too many casual romantic relationships. I do remember the fallout. We were always there for him when things went awry for whatever reason. But Rosie and Art were dedicated to each other the last three and a half years. He even had a trip planned for all of us in the fall of this year to Belgium, which was mapped out to the last detail with non-refundable tickets and was his last statement of defiance.

Art was the brother I never had. I think we were there for each other. His kindness and generosity led to my being a better psychologist and person. I would have done almost anything for him and him for me. I feel a void for his absence in my life, a feeling that many of us have now that he has left this reality forever. He was a man and a psychologist for the ages. May whatever is next be full of wonder, my good friend and brother.

Index